MEDICAL DEVICES AND EQUIPMENT

CT SCANS

PROCEDURES, APPLICATIONS AND HEALTH RISKS

MEDICAL DEVICES AND EQUIPMENT

Additional books in this series can be found on Nova's website under the Series tab.

Additional E-books in this series can be found on Nova's website under the E-book tab.

MEDICAL DEVICES AND EQUIPMENT

CT SCANS

PROCEDURES, APPLICATIONS AND HEALTH RISKS

VINCENT E. PERKEL
AND
BORIS K. SEGOVIA
EDITORS

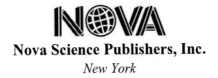

Nova Science Publishers, Inc.
New York

Copyright © 2012 by Nova Science Publishers, Inc.

All rights reserved. No part of this book may be reproduced, stored in a retrieval system or transmitted in any form or by any means: electronic, electrostatic, magnetic, tape, mechanical photocopying, recording or otherwise without the written permission of the Publisher.

For permission to use material from this book please contact us:
Telephone 631-231-7269; Fax 631-231-8175
Web Site: http://www.novapublishers.com

NOTICE TO THE READER

The Publisher has taken reasonable care in the preparation of this book, but makes no expressed or implied warranty of any kind and assumes no responsibility for any errors or omissions. No liability is assumed for incidental or consequential damages in connection with or arising out of information contained in this book. The Publisher shall not be liable for any special, consequential, or exemplary damages resulting, in whole or in part, from the readers' use of, or reliance upon, this material. Any parts of this book based on government reports are so indicated and copyright is claimed for those parts to the extent applicable to compilations of such works.

Independent verification should be sought for any data, advice or recommendations contained in this book. In addition, no responsibility is assumed by the publisher for any injury and/or damage to persons or property arising from any methods, products, instructions, ideas or otherwise contained in this publication.

This publication is designed to provide accurate and authoritative information with regard to the subject matter covered herein. It is sold with the clear understanding that the Publisher is not engaged in rendering legal or any other professional services. If legal or any other expert assistance is required, the services of a competent person should be sought. FROM A DECLARATION OF PARTICIPANTS JOINTLY ADOPTED BY A COMMITTEE OF THE AMERICAN BAR ASSOCIATION AND A COMMITTEE OF PUBLISHERS.

Additional color graphics may be available in the e-book version of this book.

Library of Congress Cataloging-in-Publication Data

CT scans : procedures, applications, and health risks / editors, Vincent E. Perkel and Boris K. Segovia.
   p. ; cm.
  Includes bibliographical references and index.
  ISBN 978-1-62100-319-9 (hardcover)
  I. Perkel, Vincent E. II. Segovia, Boris K.
  [DNLM: 1. Tomography, X-Ray Computed--methods. 2. Tomography, X-Ray Computed--adverse effects. WN 206]
  LC classification not assigned
  616.07'5722--dc23

2011032589

Published by Nova Science Publishers, Inc. † New York

CONTENTS

Preface		**vii**
Chapter 1	CT-Guided Radiofrequency Ablation of Liver Tumors *Gerlig Widmann and Reto Bale*	**1**
Chapter 2	Cardiac Computed Tomography Imaging: An update on Procedures, Applications and Health Risks *Ali Ahmad, John F. Heitner and Igor Mamkin*	**79**
Chapter 3	NeurodiagnosticPitfalls of CT Scan from Neurosurgical Viewpoint: A Personal Perspective *Bing H. Tang*	**109**
Chapter 4	Neurodiagnostic Pitfalls of CT Scans from Neuroradiological Viewpoint: A Personal Perspective *Bing H Tang and Eve Tiu*	**147**
Chapter 5	3D-CT in Oral and Maxillofacial Research *R. M. Yáñez-Vico, D. Torres-Lagares, A. Iglesias-Linares, D. González-Padilla, E. Solano-Reina and J. L. Gutierrez-Pérez*	**173**
Chapter 6	Overdenture Construction of Implants Directionally Placed Using CT Scanning Techniques *Timothy F. Kosinski*	**197**

Index 213

PREFACE

Computed tomography (CT) is an imaging technique that has revolutionized medical imaging. It is widely available, fast, and provides a detailed view of the internal organs and structures. In this book, the authors present current research in the study of the procedures, applications and health risks of CT scans. Topics included in this compilation include CT-guided radiofrequency ablation of liver tumors; cardiac CT imaging; the neurodiagnostic pitfalls of CT scanning from a neurological viewpoint; 3D-CT in oral and maxillofacial research and overdenture construction of implants using CT scanning techniques.

Chapter 1 - Image-guided percutaneous radiofrequency ablation (RFA) is increasingly used for local therapy of primary and metastatic liver tumors. Treatment success depends on the accurate planning, guidance and control of the procedure in order to ablate the tumor including a safety margin of healthy tissue and to exclude puncture related complications and thermal collateral damage.

The principles and technical considerations of RFA are explained. Different RF electrode designs and application modes are presented. Patient selection criteria and approaches are highlighted. The role and limitations of ultrasound (US)- and magnetic resonance (MR)-guided RFA, conventional computed tomography (CT)-guided and CT-fluoroscopy are discussed. Laser-guidance devices and puncture devices can improve CT-guided RF electrode placement. Virtual sonography allows fusing pre-interventional CT-scans to the sonographic images in real-time. To ablate large and irregularly shaped lesions as well as lesions located subcapsular or close to major vessels, CT-guided 3D-navigated stereotactic techniques have been introduced. Different navigation systems, image-to-patient registration techniques, stereotactic aiming devices, and medical robots are available. Patient immobilization techniques and methods for respiratory motion control are demonstrated. Post-interventional follow up imaging is essential to verify treatment success. CT protocols and radiographic signs of successful ablation necrosis, residual tumor tissue and local tumor progression are discussed.

Chapter 2 - Computed tomography (CT) is an imaging technique that has revolutionized medical imaging: it is widely available, fast, and provides a detailed view of the internal organs and structures. There are two types of CT scanners available, the conventional step and shoot (axial) and the helical CT. Axial CT is used for high resolution imaging of the lungs, coronary calcium scoring, and prospective ECG-gated coronary angiography. The two main components of CT scanners are the x-ray tube and a diametrically opposed array of detectors. The X-ray tube rotates around the patient and generates an X-ray beam and the detectors concurrently record the radiation that traverses the body while rejecting the scattered radiation emanating from outside the X-ray tube focal spot (the area of the target of the X-ray tube).

The introduction of multislice CT was a major technical advance in helical CT scanning. During multislice helical CT, a cone shaped X-ray beam (wider collimation than the conventional fan shaped X-ray beam) strikes many of the detector rows (4-320) that are arranged in parallel along the longitudinal axis (i.e., along the direction of the table motion. (Figure 1) The combination of a cone shaped X-ray beam and multiple rows of detectors allow a larger proportion of the X-ray beam to be used for imaging; multiple channels extract the data that are obtained simultaneously from different anatomic sections.

Chapter 3 - CT scanning, also being called as CAT scanning, is a noninvasive medical test that helps physicians diagnose and treat medical conditions. It combines special x-ray equipment with sophisticated computers to produce multiple images or pictures of the inside of the body. These cross-sectional images of the area being studied can then be examined on a computer monitor, printed or transferred to a compact disc, so-called CD, including internal organs, bones, soft tissue and blood vessels provide greater clarity and reveal more details than regular x-ray exams. Radiologists can more easily diagnose problems such as cancers, cardiovascular disease, infectious disease, appendicitis, trauma and musculoskeletal disorders. It is invaluable in diagnosing and treating spinal problems and injuries to the hands, feet and other skeletal structures because it can clearly show even very small bones as well as surrounding tissues such as muscle and blood vessels. As to the CT scan diagnosis of blood vessel diseases, it is very complex for Central Nervous System. There are diagnostic pitfalls of CT scans in this System.

Preface

Chapter 4 - CT scanning, also being called as CAT scanning, is a noninvasive medical test that helps physicians diagnose and treat medical conditions. It combines special x-ray equipment with sophisticated computers to produce multiple images or pictures of the inside of the body. These cross-sectional images of the area being studied can then be examined on a computer monitor, printed or transferred to a CD. CT scans of internal organs, bones, soft tissue and blood vessels provide greater clarity and reveal more details than regular x-ray exams. Radiologists can more easily diagnose problems such as cancers, cardiovascular disease, infectious disease, appendicitis, trauma and musculoskeletal disorders. It is invaluable in diagnosing and treating brain and spinal problems and injuries to the hands, feet and other skeletal structures because it can clearly show even very small bones as well as surrounding tissues such as muscle and blood vessels. As to the CT scan diagnosis of blood vessel diseases, it is very complex for Central Nervous System. There are diagnostic pitfalls of CT scans in this System. Hence, such a discussion posted in this article will be carried out from Neuroradiological viewpoint.

Chapter 5 - The arrival of the digital image to the oral and maxillofacial world has led to new research fields arising which are focused on the diagnostic potential of image manipulation in radiography. Many of those proposals have resulted in valuable tools that increase the diagnostic utility. However, many digital images have the same limitations as those found in conventional cephalometric analyses including magnification, distortion and superimposition of anatomical structures.

The analysis of the craniofacial complex has improved recently with the development of three-dimensional image technology, since we are able to observe any one of the craniofacial bones from different angles using the three-dimensional images obtained from computed tomography. Technology using 3D image provides a very effective tool for evaluating, characterizing, and drawing up the surgical treatment plan for potential orthognathic surgery patients.

An important advancement in computed tomography (CT) technology came thanks to Herman and Liu. In 1977, who presented three-dimensional reconstructions from axial slides. This method meant that it was no longer necessary to create mental three-dimensional images from two-dimensional data (those from conventional X-ray machines and from axial CT scanners), which is often inaccurate or even impossible.

The CT enables us to ascertain an exact image of the anatomical structures in three dimensions and to visualize both the soft tissues and the skeletal structures in 3D, thus improving the preparatory planning of many surgical procedures.

A new generation of compact CT scanners has been developed, specially designed for use in the head and neck region. These ultra-compact CT scanners employ cone beam geometry (cone beam - CBCT) which uses X-ray photons much more efficiently. The x-ray dose is lower in the CBCT and conventional images such as panoramic, lateral and anterior/posterior radiographs can be obtained from it. Nevertheless, three-dimensional images mean new changes and they must be interpreted in a new different way in order to extract the most information possible for the diagnosis, planning and simulation of the treatment.

Chapter 6 - CT scanning software is fast becoming a viable tool in the diagnosing of dental implant position and placement. Minimally invasive procedures may be requested by patients to reduce their anxiety and increase treatment acceptance rates. In areas where contours and width and height of bone are difficult to determine with conventional radiographic techniques, the CT scanning software allows diagnostic determination if bone quantity and quality exists and can be used to virtually place dental implants using the computer program prior to any surgical intervention. This is an outstanding tool in discussing the risks involved in surgical implant procedures and can help visualize the case finished before ever starting. Used in critical anatomic situations and for placing the implant in an ideal position in bone, CT scanning software eliminates possible manual placement errors and matches planning to prosthetic requirements. This innovative tool makes surgical placement of implants less invasive and more predictable. Prosthetic reconstruction is thus made simpler since the implants are appropriately positioned to allow for fabrication of the final prosthesis.

In: CT Scans
Editors: V. E. Perkel et al.

ISBN 978-1-62100-319-9
©2012 Nova Science Publishers, Inc.

Chapter 1

CT-GUIDED RADIOFREQUENCY ABLATION OF LIVER TUMORS

Gerlig Widmann and Reto Bale

Department of Microinvasive Therapy, Department of Radiology, Medical University of Innsbruck, Austria

ABSTRACT

Image-guided percutaneous radiofrequency ablation (RFA) is increasingly used for local therapy of primary and metastatic liver tumors. Treatment success depends on the accurate planning, guidance and control of the procedure in order to ablate the tumor including a safety margin of healthy tissue and to exclude puncture related complications and thermal collateral damage.

The principles and technical considerations of RFA are explained. Different RF electrode designs and application modes are presented. Patient selection criteria and approaches are highlighted. The role and limitations of ultrasound (US)- and magnetic resonance (MR)-guided RFA, conventional computed tomography (CT)-guided and CT-fluoroscopy are discussed. Laser-guidance devices and puncture devices can improve CT-guided RF electrode placement. Virtual sonography allows fusing pre-interventional CT-scans to the sonographic images in real-time. To ablate large and irregularly shaped lesions as well as lesions located subcapsular or close to major vessels, CT-guided 3D-navigated stereotactic techniques have been introduced. Different navigation systems, image-to-patient registration techniques, stereotactic aiming devices, and medical robots are available. Patient immobilization techniques and methods for respiratory motion control are demonstrated. Post-interventional follow up imaging is essential to verify treatment success. CT protocols and radiographic signs of successful ablation necrosis, residual tumor tissue and local tumor progression are discussed.

INTRODUCTION

In recent years, percutaneous image-guided Radiofrequency Ablation (RFA) has gained increasing importance in the medical field and has been established as an essential therapeutic option in primary and metastatic liver disease. Electrodes / probes are inserted into the tumor under image-guidance (1-4). The tumor is subsequently devitalized by thermal ablation and can be destroyed without open resection.

n contrast to resection which shows a morbidity of 15-45% and mortality of 1-5% (5-7), RFA appeared to be a relatively low risk procedure (8). Major complications that require intervention such as intraperitoneal bleeding, liver abscess, intestinal perforation, pneumothorax and haemothorax, or bile duct injury are in the range of 2–3% (8-10). The procedure related mortality rate is below 1% (8-10). Minor complications and side effects are in the range of 5–9% and may include the self-limiting post-ablation syndrome (fever up to 38.5°C, weakness, fatigue, leucocytosis) a few days after treatment (8-10). Most RFA interventions require only one overnight stay in the hospital, depending on medical comorbidities, lesion size and locations.

The attractiveness of RFA is based on the following:

- Local tumor therapy with curative intent
- Parenchym sparing ablation
- Minimal invasive percutaneous procedure
- No/minimal blood loss
- Short hospital stay.

Currently, percutaneous RFA is considered the first-line treatment for unresectable hepatocellular carcinoma (HCC) with a diameter of less than 5 cm (11). In addition, it may be considered as an alternative treatment for resectable HCC sized less than or equal to 3 cm, (11-12). It has become widespread to treat patients on the waiting list for transplantation with RFA, to downstage HCC to make patients eligible for transplantation, or to decrease HCC recurrence after liver transplantation (13-15).

Further, it has become an attractive local therapy for liver metastases from colorectal cancer (CRC) or breast cancer (16-18). More recently, it has been successfully used for treatment of intrahepatic cholangiocellular carcinoma (ICC) (19-20).

For 1-3 HCCs sized < 3 cm, complete ablation could be achieved in 96-100% of patients (21-24). A single HCC sized < 5 cm was completely ablated in 91% of patients (25). In patients with early-stage HCC who underwent percutaneous RFA, 1, 3 and 5 years survival rates of 92-100%, 49-91%, and 31-77% were published (26-31).

Local recurrence rates of liver metastases treated by RFA were in the range of 6-39%, with recurrence rates of less than 10% using newer RFA technology (32-33). After RFA for hepatic metastases from colorectal cancer, 1, 3, and 5 years survival rates were 79-96%, 28-68%, and 22-30% (16, 34-37). Using the latest RF technology with careful patient selection, local control rates and overall survival similar to that of surgical resection may be achieved (18, 38).

PRINCIPLES AND TECHNICAL CONSIDERATIONS OF RFA

The high-frequency alternating current (200–1200 KHz) from the RF electrode generates marked agitation of the ions in the tissue that immediately surrounds the uninsulated tip of the probe (Figure 1). The frictional heat produces a thermal coagulation necrosis of the surrounding tissues (1-4). To achieve an effective thermal necrosis of the tumor, 60-100 °C (degrees of Celsius) have to be achieved and maintained throughout the entire target volume for at least 4-6 minutes (Figure 2).

Due to slow thermal conduction from the electrode surface through the tissue the duration of application may increase to 10–30 minutes (2, 39). Roughly, the size of ablation correlates with the intensity and duration of RF energy deposition and the diameter of local coagulation necrosis is a function of the local mean temperature (40-42). However, the size of ablation does not increase linearly to the time of ablation and asymptotically approaches a constant ablation diameter (43). Thermal energy liberated by the electrode is dissipated radially by conduction and the temperature of the surrounding tissue diminishes exponentially with increasing distance from the electrode depending on tissue characteristics such as electrical and thermal conductivity and tissue perfusion (40, 43-45) (Figure 3).

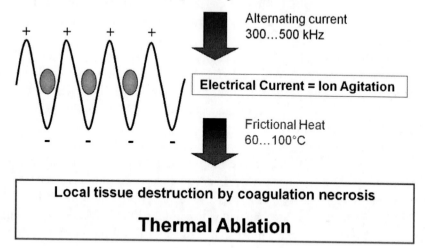

Figure 1. Principles of RFA Part1. Courtesy of A. Rogan.

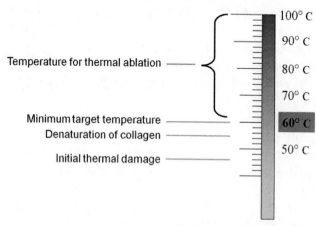

Figure 2. Principles of RFA Part 2. Courtesy of A. Rogan.

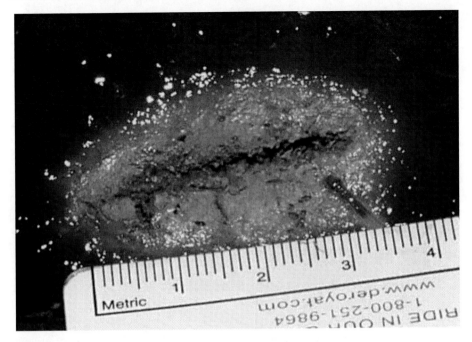

Figure 3. RF ablation necrosis in the ex-vivo liver. Central "white zone" shows tissue necrosis. Peripheral "pink zone" shows thermally altered but viable tissue.

In RFA of small HCC, the size of ablation necrosis can be larger within the tumor than in the surrounding cirrhotic liver tissue (46-47). This phenomeon has been named *"oven effect"* and was first described by Livraghi et al. (46). Typical HCC is a highly vascularized lesion similar to a sponge and the surrounding cirrhotic liver is composed of dense and fibrous tissue which acts as a shell insulating the heat and leading to a temperature increase inside the nodule. On the contrary, the *"oven effect"* may limit heat diffusion from the tumor into satellite lesions of HCC interposed by peritumoral fibrotic tissue (46-48).

Due to perfusion-mediated tissue cooling (vascular flow) in living tissue, the threshold for coagulation necrosis is 8.5°C higher than for in vitro specimens and the size and shape of coagulation necrosis around the electrodes are smaller and less uniform, respectively (45). The flowing blood in larger vessels bordering the region of RFA can cause irregularly shaped, smaller than predicted lesions with growth of residual perivascular tumor, a phenomenon named *"heat sink effect"* (3, 44-45). The size of the ablation necrosis is related to the size of the tumor being treated and this may be explained by the differences in hepatic and tumor perfusion (40, 45, 49).

ELECTRODE DESIGN

Plain Electrodes

Plain electrodes are needle-like probes with an insulated shaft and an active tip that ranges from 0.7 to 4 cm (50). The obtained RFA necrosis of a single plain electrode has an ellipsoid shape, symmetrically distributed around the electrode with the long axis depending on the length of the electrode (42, 51-52). The short axis diameter in-vivo is limited to 1.2 cm (64). For RFA in the liver, plain electrodes have been replaced by cooled electrodes.

Expandable Electrodes

Expandable electrodes contain curved needles or umbrella shaped retractable electrodes (prongs or tines) which can be extended from the central cannula after placement in the tumor (4, 50, 53-55). By expansion, the size of the metal electrode surface can be increased to up to 5 cm (50) (Figure 4).

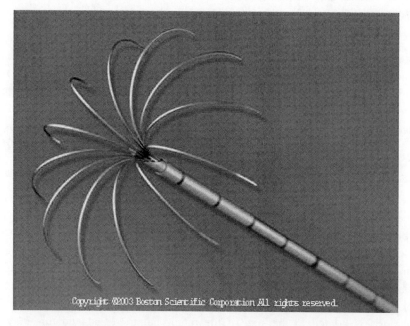

Figure 4. Expendable RF electrodes. Courtesy of Boston Scientific.

Compared to plain electrodes, the expandable electrodes create rather large, spherical or conical shaped lesions depending on the size of the electrode surface (2-3, 50-51, 56-58) (see Table 1). In-vivo, coagulation volumes of multitine electrodes were less reproducible than those induced with plain cluster electrodes (55). The multitine electrodes are more sensitive to surrounding tissue properties such as the heat sink effect and prongs located near or in vessel may lead to an irregular temperature or impedance profile, which can lead to incomplete fusion of thermal zones between the prongs (52). Potential danger of damage to vessels, bile ducts, liver capsule, surgical staples, pleura, etc., during expansion of the electrodes in lesions close to those critical structures have been described (3, 59-62). Compared to smaller-gauge plain electrodes, the larger-gauge expandable electrodes produced severe pain and intraperitoneal haemorrhage was significantly more frequently observed (61).

Table 1. Expendable monoplar electrodes. Transversal coagulation diameters

	design	size	perfused	power	duration	coagulation size (Mean +/- SD in cm)	in/ex-vivo
Miao et al. Eur Radiol 2001 (53)	3-tine curved	3 cm	N	50 W	10 min	3,3 +/- 0,3 cm	ex-vivo
				90 W		2,0 +/- 0,2 cm	
			1mL/min, 15% NaCl	50 W	10 min	5,3 +/- 0,4 cm	
				90 W		6,0 +/- 1,0 cm	
Bruners et al. Cardiovasc Intervent Radiol 2007 (54)	10-tine umbrella	3 cm	N	200W	8 min	3.0 +/- 0,1 cm	ex-vivo
			2 mL, 0,9% NaCl		10 min	3,7 +/- 0,2 cm	
Pereira et al. Radiology 2004 (55)	9-tine curved	5 cm	N	150 W	21 min	2,7 +/- 0,8 cm	in-vivo
	12-tine umbrella	4 cm	N	200 W	14 min	3,4 +/- 0,2 cm	
Denys et al. Eur Radiol 2003 (51)	9-tine curved	5 cm	N	150 W	25 min	4,6 +/- 0,5 cm	ex-vivo
						4,2 +/- 0,2 cm	in-vivo
	12-tine umbrella	4 cm	N	200 W	17 min	4,5 +/- 0,5 cm	ex-vivo
						4,3 +/- 0,5 cm	in-vivo

Cooled Electrodes

In experimental studies, tip temperatures between 45 and 55°C resulted in charring which insulates surrounding tissue from further ablation (41, 63). Cooled electrodes contain an internal chamber of the probe that is perfused of cold saline of 0-8°C at 10 – 25 mL/min. (50) (Figure 5).

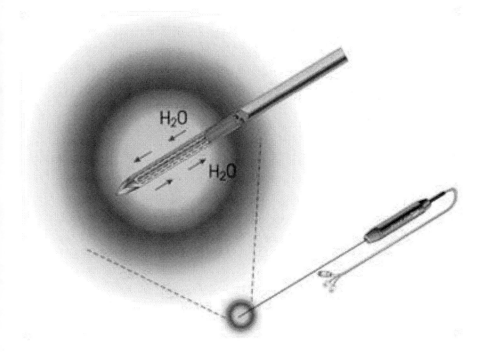

Figure 5. Cooled RF electrodes. Courtesy of Covidien.

The cooling permits greater energy deposition in tissues resulting in greater heating at distant to the electrode and a greater coagulation diameter (2, 40, 45, 50) (see Tables 2, 3). In-vivo, cooled electrodes resulted in a decrease of tip temperature to 25-35°C (41, 64). 65 W for 12 min could be applied without inducing charring and produced a lesion diameter of 2.4 cm. By comparison, without internal cooling only a maximum of 20 W could be deposited, resulting in only a 1.2 cm RFA lesion (64). Simultaneous use of non-cooled monopolar probes at interprobe distance of 1.5 cm or less in ex-vivo liver produced uniform tissue necrosis, while at interprobe distance of 2 cm or more, independent lesions with incomplete necrosis between probes were obtained (65).

Table 2. Plain monopolar electrodes. Transversal coagulation diameters

	cooled	perfused	mode	spacing (number of electrodes/cm of spacing)	power	duration	coagulation size (Mean +/- SD)	in/ex-vivo
Goldberg et al. Radiology 1998 (80)	Y	N	single		150 W	45 min	2,7 +/- 0,2 cm	ex-vivo
						12 min	1,8 +/- 0,1 cm	in-vivo
Denys et al. Eur Radiol 2003 (51)	N	1,7mL/min 0,9% NaCl	single		50 W	15 min	4,6 +/- 0,6 cm	ex-vivo
							3,4 +/- 0,8 cm	in-vivo
Ni et al. Eur Radiol 2000 (67)	Y	1mL/min 5,0% NaCl	single		50 W	10 min	4,9 +/- 0,6 cm	ex-vivo
					90 W		6,6 +/- 0,9 cm	
					90 W		4,2 +/- 0,4 cm	in-vivo
					150 W		5,2 +/- 1.0 cm	
Lee et al. Koren J Radiol 2004a (72)	Y	N	single		200 W	10 min	2,6 +/- 0,3 cm	ex-vivo
	N	2mL/min, 6,0% NaCL					2,7 +/- 0,7 cm	
	Y	2mL/min, 6,0% NaCL					4,9 +/- 0,4 cm	
Lee et al. Korean J Radiol 2004b (69)	Y	11mL, 5% NaCl	single		200 W	10 min	2,2 +/- 0,3 cm	ex-vivo

Table 2. (Continued)

		1mL/min, 5,0% NaCl					5,2 +/- 0,6 cm	
		6 mL, 36% NaCl					4,2 +/- 0,5 cm	
		0,5mL/min, 36,0% NaCl					5,4 +/- 0,4 cm	
Laeseke et al. Radiology 2006 (83)	Y	N	single		200 W	12 min	1,6 +/- 0,6 cm (min)	in-vivo
							2,0 +/- 0,5 cm (max)	
						16 min	1,7 +/- 0,5 cm (min)	
							2,2 +/- 0,6 cm (max)	
			cluster	3/2 cm		12 min	2,1 +/- 0,5 cm (min)	
							2,9 +/- 0,3 cm (max)	
						16 min	2,3 +/- 0,3 cm (min)	
							3,2 +/- 0,4 cm (max)	
			switching	3/2 cm		12 min	2,8 +/- 0,6 cm (min)	
							4,2 +/- 0,7 cm (max)	
						16 min	3,2 +/- 0,6 cm (min)	
							4,2 +/- 0,6 cm (max)	
Lee et al. Invest Radiol 2007a (82)	Y	N	overlapping	3/3 cm	200 W	36 min	5,3 +/- 0,3 cm (min)	ex-vivo
							5,5 +/- 0,2 cm (max)	
			switching	3/3 cm		12 min	5,0 +/- 0,4 cm (min)	
							5,3 +/- 0,3 cm (max)	

Table 2. (Continued)

			switching	3/2 cm		12 min	4,6 +/- 0,5 cm (min)	in-vivo
							4,8 +/- 0,3 cm (max)	
			switching	3/3 cm		12 min	4,8 +/- 0,8 cm (min)	
							5,2 +/- 0,5 cm (max)	

Table 3. Plain bipolar electrodes. Transversal coagulation diameters
(c-monopolar – consecutive monopolar; s-monopolar – simultaneous monopolar)

	cooled	perfused	mode	spacing (number of electrodes/cm of spacing)	power	duration	coagulation size (Mean +/- SD)	in/ex-vivo
Clasen et al. Radiology 2006 (87)	Y	N	multipolar	3/2 cm	100W	19 min	4,5 +/- 0,3 cm	ex-vivo
					125 W	9 min	4,2 +/- 0,7 cm	
				3/3 cm	100 W	22 min	5,2 +/- 0,3 cm	
					125 W	12 min	4,9 +/- 0,7 cm	
				3/4 cm	100 W	27 min	6,1 +/- 0,7 cm	
					125 W	16 min	5,5 +/- 0,3 cm	
Lee et al. Invest Radiol 2007b (91)	Y	N	multipolar	3/2 cm	250 W	18 min	4,3 +/- 0,8 cm (min)	in-vivo
							5,2 +/- 1,2 cm (max)	

Table 3. (Continued)

Lee et al. Korean J Radiol 2006 (90)	Y	2mL/min, 6,0% NaCl	c-monopolar	3/4 cm	150 W	36 min	2,7 +/- 0,1 cm (max)	ex-vivo
							2,4 +/- 0,2 cm (min)	
			s-monopolar	3/4 cm	150 W	20 min	5,7 +/- 0,7 cm (max)	
							3,5 +/- 1,0 cm (min)	
			multipolar	3/3 cm	150 W	20 min	4,6 +/- 0,4 cm (max)	
							4,3 +/- 0,3 cm (min)	
				3/4 cm			5,7 +/- 0,7 cm (max)	
							5,3 +/- 0,4 cm (min)	
				3/5 cm			6,0 +/- 0,5 cm (max)	
							3,7 +/- 0,9 cm (min)	
			multipolar	3/4 cm	150 W	20 min	6,5 +/- 0,2 cm (max)	in-vivo
							3,7 +/- 0,8 cm (min)	

Wet (Perfused) Electrodes

Pretreatment bolus injection of saline (saline enhanced RFA) can increase electrical conductivity of the tissue and thus may increase the thermal necrosis (1, 48, 53, 66-69) (see Tables 1, 2). Saline enhanced RFA created lesions of 1.4 cm +/- 0.1, in ex-vivo liver, and 1.2 cm +/- 0.1 in in-vivo animal liver, while without saline enhancement, lesion sizes were 1.0 +/- 0.2, and 0.8 +/- 0.1 cm, respectively (70).

Based on these findings, wet electrodes have been designed that have openings at the tip or along the electrode for perfusion of 0.9-36% saline solution at a rate of 0.5-2 mL/min during ablation (50, 69, 71-72) (Figure 6). In all electrode designs, wet RFA provided significant larger mean ablation volumes than that obtained with dry ablation or a pretreatment saline injection (53-54, 69, 71-75) (see Tables 1-3). Saline perfusion is superior to pretreatment saline bolus, probably due to the increased generator output that is achieved by tissue cooling and the diffusion of boiling saline into the tissue (69-70). Significant larger short-axis diameter of coagulation necrosis were obtained with 6 % saline compared to 0.9 % saline solution, however, concentration of saline above 6 % did not further increase the extent of coagulation necrosis (76). Perfusion rates of 2mL/min produced significantly larger necrosis than 0.5 mL/min (76).

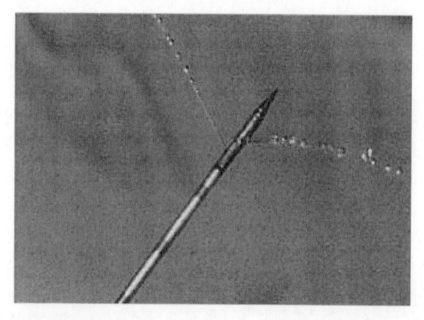

Figure 6. Wet (perfused) electrodes.

CT-Guided Radiofrequency Ablation of Liver Tumors

A drawback of the saline perfusion technique is the concern for an irregular shape of coagulation necrosis due to uneven distribution of injected saline (66, 77-78). There is increased risk of thermal injury to adjacent organs or portal thrombosis related to diffusion of hot saline along vessels, the needle track and the liver capsule (51-52, 76). Concerns about the potential risk of liver tissue injury-related toxicity of saline when large amounts of saline are perfused into normal parenchyma have been reported (69, 76). Furthermore there is a theoretical concern that saline contaminated with viable tumor cells may leak out of the electrode track and causes peritoneal or track seeding (69).

ABLATION MODES

Monopolar RFA Systems

In monopolar systems the radiofrequency current flows from the generator through the noninsulated tip of the probe into the tissue and follows the natural paths in the soft tissue towards a large dispersive electrode (grounding pad) to form a closed-loop electric circuit (50-51, 69, 72) (Figure 7). To disperse equal amounts of energy and heat and to prevent skin burns at the grounding pad sites multiple large dispersive electrodes are applied (39, 79).

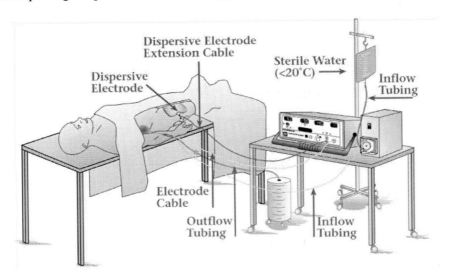

Figure 7. Monopolar RFA systems. Courtesy of Covidien.

During the ablation cycle, the generator's impedance feedback system senses maximum energy deposition into the lesion and uses pulsing to keep the energy output at its optimal level.

Monopolar systems are available for every electrode design (see Table 1 and 2). Single cooled monopolar electrodes produced maximal coagulation of 2.9 cm in ex vivo liver and 1.8 cm in in-vivo liver (80). Three separate cooled monopolar electrodes and simultaneous RF application to electrode clusters spaced 0.5 cm apart produced of RFA necrosis with short axis diameters of 4.7 cm +/- 0.1 in ex-vivo liver and 3.1 cm +/- 0.2 cm in in-vivo liver (80).

Multiple electrode ablation based on 3 cooled monopolar electrodes and a rapid-switching multi-electrode control allows physicians to simultaneously treat multiple tumors, which substantially reduces procedure time and anesthesia risk. An in-vivo model showed that such a system was able to simultaneously create three separate ablation zones of equivalent size compared with single-electrode controls (81). Ex-vivo, there was no significant difference in the mean ablation volume using three switching monopolar electrodes placed at 3 cm interprobe distance compared to overlapping conventional monopolar RFA (82). An in-vivo study in 15 pigs comparing switching multiple electrode RFA (three electrodes at 2 cm inter-probe distance) to cluster RFA showed that the obtained coagulation necrosis was significantly larger for the switching multiple probe RFA with minimum diameter, 3.2 cm vs 2.3 cm; maximum diameter, 4.2 cm vs 3.2 cm; volume, 29.1 cm(3) vs. 13.1 cm(3) (83). In-vivo, 3 cooled monopolar electrodes at 2 cm inter-probe distance produced areas of well-defined coagulation with a volume and short-axis coagulation diameter of 35.5 +/- 5.7cm(3) and 4.6 +/- 0.5 cm, and at 3 cm inter-probe distance 40.7 +/- 12.8(3) cm and 4.8 +/- 0.8 cm, respectively (82). The circularity (isometric ratio) decreases with increasing interprobe diameter and showed 0.95 at 2 cm interprobe distance and 0.85 at 3 cm. Inter-probe distance of larger than 3 cm (3.5 cm and 4 cm for 20 minutes) could not create confluent coagulation necrosis (82). (see Table 2)

Bipolar RFA Systems

In bipolar systems the radiofrequency current flows exclusively between the two poles of the electrode, thus a grounding pad is not required (50, 84-87). The radiofrequency current is controlled by a microprocessor and flows at short intervals between the pairs of electrodes. By means of microprocessor controlled evaluation of the time-dependent resistance sequence, the system determines the maximum power uptake of the tissue, adapted to the momentary treatment status, and automatically adjusts the power control unit (86-87). In a multipolar setting, currently three (max. 6) probes can be used simultaneously, the current flowing alternately between the 6 (max. 12) poles of the electrodes (86-88) (Figure 7). The presence of multiple independent heat sources leads to less heat dissipation and creates a synergistic effect of additive heat diffusion (87).

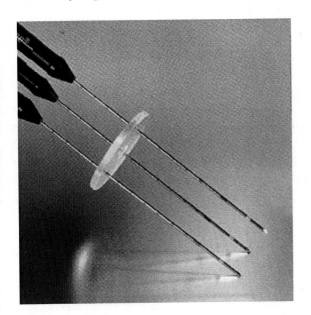
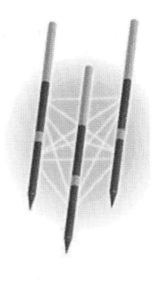

Figure 7. Multipolar RFA with three electrodes. Olympus.

The size of the necrosis depends on the power output and duration of RF energy delivery. Longer durations of energy delivery created a larger dimension of coagulation necrosis and lower maximum power output produced larger zones of coagulation but with a prolonged ablation time (76, 87).

Lee et al. (76-77, 89) compared simultaneous monopolar mode, alternating monopolar mode, or bipolar mode using saline-perfused (6% NaCl solution, 1 mL/min) cooled bipolar electrodes and a 200 W generator in an explanted bovine liver. Bipolar mode showed a more rapid increase and higher temperature between two electrodes than monopolar modes. Two cooled wet bipolar electrodes at inter-probe distance of 3 cm, produced coagulation diameters of 2.4 ± 1.2 cm in simultaneous monopolar mode, 4.5 ± 1.0 cm in alternating monopolar mode, and 6.1 ± 0.9 cm in the bipolar mode. At inter-probe distance of 5-cm, the simultaneous monopolar mode did not allow to produce a homogeneous necrosis but produced two separated ablation spheres. The alternating monopolar mode allowed for a confluent ablation but with a waist (vertical diameter of 2.9 +/- 1 cm) and only the bipolar mode produced a homogeneous single ablation area with a transversal diameter of 5.9 +/- 0.9 cm and a vertical diameter of 6.6 ± 0.4 cm (89). Using 3 cooled, wet bipolar probes, the short axis diameter of the ablation was 4.3 cm at 3 cm inter-probe distance, and 5.3 cm at 4 cm inter-probe distance. At 5 cm inter-probe distance, the short axis diameter decreased to 3.7 and the necrosis became irregular. In-vivo (pig), 3 cooled wet multipolar RFA at 150 W for 20 min. at 4 cm inter-probe spacing provided confluent necrosis with long-axis diameter of 6.5 cm, vertical diameter of 4.8 cm and short-axis diameter of 3.7 cm (90). Multiple-electrode mulipolar cooled dry RFA provided similar results when compared to cooled dry switching monopolar RFA (91). (See Table 3).

Bipolar electrodes have to be placed in equidistant and parallel position to create homogeneous, overlapping necroses (76, 88). In cases for which critical anatomic structures or obstacles such as vessels or ribs prevent parallel and equidistant positioning, the current will flow to the nearest portion of the exposed ground probes and may result in bizarrely shaped necroses (87, 90). As all the current originating from one electrode must also enter the second electrode, there is no possibility to independently control the amount of heat generated in the vicinity of each electrode. This may lead to different amounts of cooling at the location of each of the electrodes due to difference in perfusion. One electrode may reach higher temperature than the other, which can result in boiling and rapid increase of impedance (92). Since all the current flows between the electrodes, in a perfused organ, there is a lack of current density in the periphery around each probe resulting in a minimal necrosis formation outside the center of the triangle (if three electrodes are used) (90).

PATIENT SELECTION

Patient selection is essential for therapeutic success in RFA. Tumor stage, tumor size, number of tumors, and tumor location are influential factors. The decision towards RFA treatment should always be individually planned in consensus of an interdisciplinary tumor board. Conventional liver biochemical tests, prothrombin time, and complete blood cell counts are measured before treatment. Liver chirrosis classified lower than Child-Pugh class B, prothrombin time < 23 seconds, prothrombin acticity > 40% and platelet count > 40,000/mL are required for RFA therapy (9, 48, 61, 93). Patients with American Society of Anesthesiologists (ASA) score ≥ III should not be treated (94).

Even more than 5 and large (> 5 cm) liver tumors may be successfully treated with RFA (48, 88, 95). However, patients with advanced liver disease and / or with large tumors that require extensive RFA can be at risk of liver failure, thus sufficient liver remnant has to be warranted (9, 96). Patients with manifest ascites should not be treated, as the ascites may enhance the risk of intra-abdominal infection and sepsis. Pneumobilia increases the risk of abscess and sepsis, and the presence of a bilioenteric anastomosis is generally seen as a contraindication for RFA due to the increased risk of infection (9). Tumors within 1 cm close to the central bile duct are considered a contraindication (94).

PLANNING AND APPROACH

The goal of RFA is to ablate the entire tumor and a safety margin of surrounding healthy tissue. Precise planning and targeting are important to prevent technical failure (Figure 8). Movement of the target and the obstacles due to respiration have to be taken into concern.

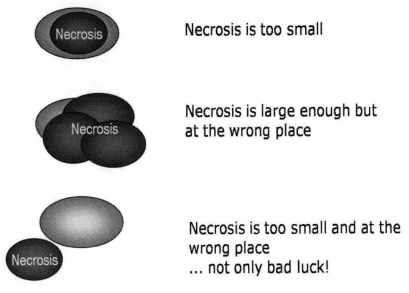

Figure 8. Imprecision leads to technical failure and local tumor progression.

When using multiple probes, it is important that the probes keep correct distance in a favourable parallel position. Further, the selection of safe trajectories from the skin entry points to the targets is essential as many different obstacles including the ribs, pleura, lung, stomach, intestine and large vessels have to be passed (Figure 9). Every probe repositioning and the final removal of the probe after RFA has to be performed in hot (70-90°C) ablation mode ("hot withdrawal" or "track ablation"), in order to prevent local hemorrhage and neoplastic seeding (9, 97).

Percutaneous image-guided RFA can be performed repeatedly under conscious sedation or general anesthesia with standard cardiac, pressure, and oxygen monitoring (48, 93, 98). Only small tumors which require one or a maximum of two probe positions may be treated under conscious sedation. For larger tumors, or multiple tumors, or when the patient is particularly anxious, general anaesthesia is recommended (48). In order to prevent postoperative pain, subcutaneous and pericapsular injection of 10 mL longlasting local anasethetic (e.g. napivacain) may be useful (16, 99). Although there are no guidelines, preoperative intravenous administration of antibiotics may be given in order to prevent possible infectious complications.

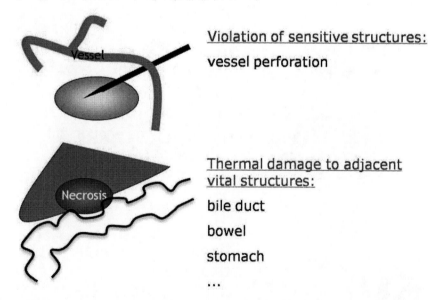

Figure 9. Imprecision leads to puncture related complications or collateral thermal damage.

Tumor Size and Shape

The issue of planning reliable tumor-ablation may be interpreted as a geometrical problem concerning both the induced necrosis as well as the spatial relationship of the necrosis to the tumor. The size of the ablation necrosis should cover the entire tumor including a safety margin of surrounding healthy tissue. For small HCC with well defined borders 0.5 cm may be sufficient, however, in HCC and metastases with poorly defined borders, 1 cm ablation margins need to be included in the planning (2-3, 49, 59, 100). Thus, the interventionalist has to consider that the diameter of the ablation must be 2 cm larger than the diameter of the tumor (3, 101-102).

Lesions sized $\geq$ 1 cm require more than one probe or several probe positions in order to treat the tumor with overlapping elipsoidal (single straight electrodes) or spherical (single expandable electrodes) ablation zones, respectively (3, 59, 95, 103). If a 1 cm tumor free margin is included, in a single ablation model, 3-, 4-, and 5 cm ablation spheres can ablate tumors measuring 1-, 2-, and 3 cm, respectively (101). If six ablation spheres are placed in orthogonal planes around a spherical tumor, the largest tumor that may be treated with a 3-cm ablation device has a diameter of 1.75 cm, whereas 4- and 5-cm ablation spheres can be used to treat tumors measuring 3 and 4.25 cm, respectively. With 14 ablation spheres, the treatable tumor size is increased to 3, 4.6, or 6.3 cm, respectively (101). Chen et al. (59, 95) proposed a mathematical protocol for RFA of spherical tumors with a 5.0 cm ablation device. A minimum of 4 ablation spheres is required for target lesions of 5.0 – 5.3 cm, 6 ablation spheres for lesions of 5.7 – 6.1 cm, 8 ablation spheres for lesions of 6.5 – 6.6 cm and 12 ablation spheres for lesions of 6.7 – 7.5 cm (59, 95). Using this mathematical model in a total of 332 patients with 503 liver lesions, early necrosis rates were 95.8% for HCC and 94.9% for liver metastases, with local recurrence rates of 10.7% and 14.9%, respectively. The early necrosis rate of tumors larger than 3.5 cm was 91.3% (59).

Irregularly Shaped Lesions

Many lesions have irregular margins and satellite lesions. Therefore, irregular lesions cannot be ablated according to the basic models described above as the condition of (rather) spherically shaped volume of interest is not met. In order to achieve overlapping necrosis, the main part of the tumor can be ablated according to a spherical tumor protocol, whereas the remaining irregular and protruding parts have to be treated with adjacent ablation spheres (59, 103).

Tumor Location

Central Tumors

Tumors adjacent or within 1 cm to the central structures of the liver include the risk of vessel perforation or thermal damage to the bile duct with bile duct stenoses or formation of biliomas (9, 96). For prevention, intra-ductal cooling by cold perfusion via a choledochal incision has been reported to allow ablation without bile duct damage (104). However, the procedure still carries the risk of biliary infection through ascending gastrointestinal bacteria.

Perfused electrodes may lead to heat diffusion along the portal vein and increase the risk of bile duct damage or lethal portal vein thrombosis and are therefore not recommended in this location (51). Expandable electrodes have to be used with extreme care in order to prevent any perforation or thermal damage related to prong expansion.

Tumors Close to Adjacent Organs

RFA of lesions within 1 cm of the liver capsule adjacent to organs carries the risk of collateral thermal damage and perforation (97). Tumors abutting the *diaphragm* may increase the risk of pneumothorax, pleural effusion, pleuritis, perforation of the diaphragm with hernia, bilio-pleural fistulas and abscess formation (62, 105). However, in most patients RFA adjacent to the diaphragm could be safely performed with symptoms of mild or moderate right shoulder pain for up to 2 weeks (62). A safety distance of 5 mm from the RF electrode tip to the diaphragm is recommended.

RFA of tumors adjacent to the *gallbladder* has proven to be safe and feasible, taking into account self limited morbidity after ablation in most patients, related to mild iatrogenic cholecystits with right-upper quadrant pain (106). Among *hollow viscera*, the colon is at greater risk than the stomach or small bowel for thermally mediated perforation (96, 107).

In order to prevent thermal injury, adjacent organs can be separated from the liver by injection of various amounts (150 to 1000 mL) of 5% glucose solution into the peritoneum (107-109), percutaneous interposition of a balloon (110) or "laparoscopic liver packing" in which prior to RFA, swabs soaked with 5% glucose are placed between liver and adjacent organs under laparoscopy and removed afterwards in the same session (Bale & Widmann, unpublished data). Other, less predictable techniques include the lifting of an extendable electrode to slightly draw the tumor away from the adjacent organ at risk and fixing the electrode shaft in position (59). As a general recommendation, electrodes should be positioned perpendicular to the critical structure. A modified Habib technique may be very helpful and allows successful devascularisation of tumors or segments (111-120). Due to the possible perforation or unfavourable prong expansion, extreme care should be taken when expandable electrodes are used (59, 62). In the critical area, multiple small ablations are preferred over large ablations (59). The key area may be alternatively treated with PEI or TACE, however, hypovascular metastases do not respond well to those therapies (93, 100, 121-122).

Tumors Close to Vessels

In the vicinity of large vessels, the associated cooling effects with a higher probability for recurrence have to be counteracted (3, 41, 44-45). It is recommended to place the electrodes and thus the central part of the developing necrosis as close as achievable to the vessel without damaging it (19, 86, 103, 123). When the tumor feeding vessel is visible, the area of the tumor where the feeding vessel enters should be ablated first. This can reduce the negative effects of vascularisation associated tissue cooling (59). If the tumor has direct contact to or invades major hepatic veins, perioperative administration of 5.000 I.E. of Heparin may prevent pulmonary embolism. Expandable electrodes may not be placed as close as plain electrodes and increase the risk of vascular damage during extension of the prongs (3). Further, incomplete necrosis between the prongs due to higher sensitivity for cooling effects may occur (52). For these reasons, expandable electrodes cannot be recommended in this tumor location.

Subcapsular Tumors

Subcapsular lesions have an increased risk of local recurrence (47, 124). It is important that the liver capsule that overlies the tumor closer than 1 cm is included in the RF necrosis (93, 125). Precise targeting may be difficult for tumors between the anterior and posterior liver capsules, such as in the inferior angle of the right lobe, or the left lateral segments (3). In order to avoid bleeding and tumor spread through the perforated capsule, the tumor should be targeted through non-tumorous tissue and a careful track ablation has to be performed (97, 126). Wet electrodes may lead to unintended diffusion of hot saline along the needle track with thermal damage to the liver capsule and adjacent areas and are not recommended in this location (51). Subcapsular lesions should be carefully treated using an expandable electrode (47, 96, 126-127).

US AND MR-GUIDED RFA

Ultrasound (US)

Image Guidance

US is the most commonly used method for guidance of RF treatment (3, 93, 100, 122). The big advantages are the low costs, absence of ionizing radiation, potential to choose arbitrary puncture trajectories and the real time visualization of the probe during advancement. However, lesions in the liver dome and deeply located lesions may sometimes be difficult to localize. In approximately half of the patients the requested RFA procedure is not feasible, mainly due to inconspicuous tumors at planning sonography (55.8%), and an inadequate electrode path (23.9%) (128). To improve the sonic window and electrode path in lesions in the liver dome, generation of an artificial ascites may displace the liver downward (127, 129).

In progressive cirrhosis, the echogenity of the parenchyma becomes heterogeneous and some HCCs may not be visualized or differentiated from regenerative nodules (130). In liver metastases, borders are frequently not clear on B-mode US due to the lack of a tumor capsule and cellular infiltration of the metastatic lesions (131). Plain electrodes can be usually well delineated on US, however, due to the relatively low resolution and contrast, the position of the retractable curved tines of a multitined expandable electrode may not accurately be confirmed by US (62).

Monitoring and Treatment Evaluation

During RFA the treated tissue appears hyperechoic due to thermal tissue changes with the presence of microbubbles from vaporization of intracellular water (*"gassing out"*) (125, 132). One has to be aware that the microbubbles do not correspond exactly to the ablation zone and may not indicate complete tumor ablation. Obscuration of the US image is particularly problematic in large tumors, when electrodes have to be repositioned to generate multiple overlapping ablation zones (125). The ablated area may be hypoechoic (59%), hyperechoic (25%) or isoechoic (16%) (133). Differentiation between tumor necrosis and residual or recurrent tumor after local ablative treatment is unreliable on B-mode US, color Doppler US and power Doppler US (2, 16, 99, 134-136). Sonographic appearance of lesions changes rapidly within 5 min after the termination of ablation (137). An early echogenic cloud becomes peripherally hypoechoic with a variable thin

CT-Guided Radiofrequency Ablation of Liver Tumors

echogenic rim. Compared to histopathology, both early US (0-2 min after ablation) and delayed US (2-5 min after ablation) lead to an underestimation of true lesion sizes (137). In cirrhotic liver, the diameter of the echogenic response correlates significantly with the mean diameter of the necrosis (correlation coefficient, 0.84); however, the echogenic response tends to overestimate the minimal diameter of necrosis and to underestimate the maximum diameter of the necrosis (138).

Contrast Enhanced US (CEUS)

Image Guidance

Last-generation US contrast agents improve the assessment of tumoral and parenchymal microcirculation. Following an intravenous slow bolus administration the Doppler signals within the macro- and microvasculatures are enhanced for several minutes due to increase of the linear backscattering from the microvascular blood pool (139-140). CEUS can improve localization and characterization of focal liver lesions that cannot be adequately detected or characterized in B-mode US (136, 141-143). In particularly difficult cases, the electrode insertion has to be performed during the specific phase in which the maximum lesion conspicuity is observed, such as in arterial phase for hypervascular lesions (HCC and hypervascular metastases) or in the portal or equilibrium phases for hypovascular metastases (144). CEUS may be difficult for tumors located deeper than 10 cm from the skin because of the decreasing power of the US beam (145-146). As a guidance modality, CEUS can significantly improve probe placement and reduce treatment sessions required (136, 147). CEUS enabled accurate targeting of liver metastases that were previously invisible with conventional US (148). In a series of 53 patients with a total of 97 liver metastases, CEUS detected tiny hypovascular metastases not noticed on contrast-enhanced helical CT in 12% of patients (144). This led to a significant modification of treatment strategy, since 38% of these patients, initially enrolled for RF ablation, were excluded due to the unexpectedly large number of metastases detected (144). A prospective randomized controlled trial showed that CEUS-guided RFA had a significant higher complete ablation rate after a single treatment session than the control group using B-mode US-guided RFA (94.7% vs. 65%) (147).

Monitoring and Treatment Evaluation

5-10 min after ablation, usually a thin and uniform enhancing rim can be found along the periphery of the ablation area (144). In order to avoid misinterpretation of residual viable tumor, the immediate postablation images have to be compared to stored preablative scans with scrutiny (144).

In the detection of HCC tumor vascularity and assessment of response to RFA after 1 month, CEUS provided results comparable to those obtained with contrast enhanced CT or MR (145, 149). In a group of 109 patients with HCC in liver cirrhosis and in 53 patients with liver metastases undergoing a single session of percutaneous RFA, the sensitivity of CEUS for the detection of residual tumor was almost equivalent to that of contrast-enhanced helical CT (150). In seventy-five patients with 81 nodular HCCs (1.3 – 4.8 cm) treated with percutaneous RFA, 10/81 (12%) showed either nodular or crescentic enhancing foci at the margins of ablation zones at CEUS, suggesting residual unablated tumors (151). Contrast-enhanced CT obtained 1 month after treatment confirmed residual unablated tumors in the same 10 lesions with a diagnostic agreement between 1-month follow-up CT and CEUS of 100% (151). When CEUS was used for detection of residual foci that were immediately treated with additional RFA in the same session until no further residual enhancement was detectable, only 5 of 51 cases (9.8%) showed a 1.2-1.9-cm residual tumor depicted at postablation CT (144). CEUS-guided additional directed therapy could drop the rate of partially unablated HCCs prior to the introduction of CEUS for real-time management of ablation for 16.1% to 5.9% (144, 148, 150).

Magnetic Resonance (MR)

Image Guidance

Due to the excellent soft-tissue contrast of MR, lesions may be detected without the use of contrast (56). However, optimal protocols include dynamic gadolinium contrast-enhanced T1-weighted sequences and additional late enhancement studies with specific contrast agents (152-156). To minimize the risk of nephrogenic systemic fibrosis, non-cyclic Gadolinum based contrast agent is contraindicated in patients with a chronic renal failure with glomerular filtration rate of less or equal to 30 ml/min/1.73m2 (157-158). Unlike CT, MR does not require ionizing radiation. Recent open-configuration scanners improve patient access, allowing treatment of the patient in the gantry (56, 159-160). For probe guidance MR has multiplanar and interactive capabilities with near real-time imaging of the target and the probe during advancement. T1-weighted 2D-FLASH

CT-Guided Radiofrequency Ablation of Liver Tumors 27

sequences allow for a clear identification of the probe based on the signal void, without significant susceptibility artefacts (161). MR imaging can be advantageously used to guide overlapping ablation by enabling a precise repositioning of the RF probe (162).

Compared to CT, MR it is more susceptible to motion artefacts and may contain noise and geometric deformation artefacts (163). The availability of interventional open MR is limited and expensive MR compatible equipment is required (56, 162, 164). Compared to high field diagnostic scanners, low field open scanners have a lower spatial resolution which limits the detection of small tumors (161). Safety protocols for interventional MR have to be engrained by training and policy enforcement. Such protocols may include scanner and intervention room configurations, operational safety rules, screening of patients to rule out contraindications for MR such as pacemakers, some aneurysm clips, metal fragments in the eye, mechanical device implants, etc. (152, 165).

Monitoring and Treatment Evaluation

MR is sensitive to thermal effects during the entire RF ablation procedure (163, 166). Quantitative MR thermometry acquired simultaneously during RFA in a pig model revealed an accurate correlation between the thermal dose and both, the white necrotic and red hypervascular zone on histologic analysis (167). Average differences between macroscopic size measurements of the white and red zone and the thermal dose predictions were 4.1 +/- 1.93 mm and -0.71 +/- 2.47 mm, with correlation values of 0.97 and 0.99, respectively (168). Monitoring of thermally induced coagulation by MR is supportive to control the ablation procedure and to prevent unintended thermal damage from critical structures surrounding the target region (163, 169).

Residual tumor appears as focal enhancement within or at the border of the treated lesion in the Gadolinium-enhanced MR (169). In contrast to CT, tissue-specific MR contrast agents such as hepatobiliary and reticuloendothelial system targeted agents can be used (153, 170-171). The advantage of these agents is that they allow distinction between healthy liver tissue and tumors and may help distinguishing residual tumor from perfusion abnormalities on late-venous images (171-173). Overestimation of the ablation success compared to histopathology has to be acknowledged (174). Using either MR or CT for evaluation of treatment success complete histologic response rates after RFA of 70% vs. radiologic response rates of 85% have been reported (149).

CT-GUIDED RFA

Contrast enhanced multi-phase CT-imaging excellently delineates liver tumors and metastases. For guidance of RFA, CT scanners with a large gantry and moveable, sliding gantries are more convenient than standard diagnostic CT scanners (123, 175-176) (Figure 10).

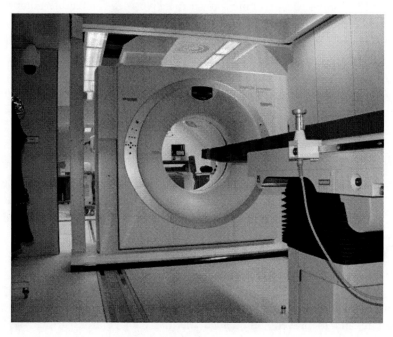

Figure 10. Sliding gantry interventional CT scanner (Siemens Somatom Sensation open) with a large gantry opening of 82 cm.

Contrast enhanced CT phases (arterial phase – high contrast in the arteries; portal phase – high contrast in the portal vein and the hepatic veins) may be necessary for optimal tumour visualization and treatment planning. After intravenous injection of 90-120 ml Iodixanol 320 mg J/mg, 3ml/sec., the arterial phase CT scans should be started under bolus tracking (contrast higher than 220 Hounsfield Units in the region of interest in the abdominal aorta) after a delay of 14 seconds. The portal phase CT scans should follow a delay of 25 seconds thereafter. A slice thickness of 3 mm can be recommended.

To improve visibility of target lesions, multimodal *image fusion* of *CT-MR-PET-SPECT* may be integrated. By fusion of an MR to the interventional CT, RFA can be performed in lesions which cannot be reliably detected by CT, or when CT-contrast media is contraindicated. Registration accuracy of CT-MR images is in the range of 1-5 mm (163). By fusion of functional images to the interventional CT images, PET or SPECT positive lesions may be selectively treated.

Image fusion can be manually performed by paired-point matching using external markers or anatomical landmarks. Alternatively registration may be automatically performed based on voxel similarity measures using joint entropy or mutual information (87). Depending on the software and workstation, an image fusion may requires up to 3-5 minutes (177). The accuracy of image fusion is influenced by physiologic motion and the non-rigid nature of organs (57, 123, 130, 175, 178-180). Different patient positioning, organ shift, change in organ shape and stomach contents during the RFA procedure compared to preinterventional imaging has to be encountered (177). Hardware based CT-PET or CT-SPECT image fusion is provided by combined scanners but is not feasible for interventional purposes.

Conventional CT Guidance

Before imaging, a radioopaque rod is placed on the skin of the patient and used to calculate the entry point of the planned trajectory on the skin. All scans should be performed in expiratory phase to compensate motions from breathing. Usually targeting is performed in the axial plane (181). If the axial plane does not provide an optimal path to the target, the CT gantry may be tilted to up to 25%. After defining target, entry, angulations and targeting depth on the planning CT, the electrode is introduced incrementally, often interrupted by sequential control scans (182-183) (Figure 11).

CT-fluoroscopy provides simultaneous needle manipulation and CT scanning (real-time method) or involves very short fluoroscopic CT scans, for checking the position of the needle (quick-check method) (181, 184-185). As a drawback, the continuous CT scanning may deliver (potentially high) radiation doses to the staff and the patient (184-187).

Many tumours are only visible after administration of contrast media and the lesion may only be seen in the contrast-enhanced planning CT and not in the native control CTs. Image fusion of the planning CT to the native control CT may improve localization during punctures that are performed under repeated unenhanced control images (177). However, in patients with severe contrast media allergy, underlying renal disease or inability to tolerate multiple intravenous contrast doses, CT-guidance may be very difficult (56, 188).

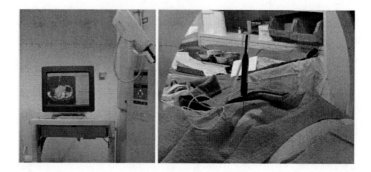

Figure 11. Conventional CT-guided RFA. Left – CT monitor with the axial control images. Right – RF needle placed in the liver of the patient.

Guidance Devices

To improve CT-guided punctures in terms of reduction of needle passes and control CT-scans, *laser guidance devices* have been implemented in clinical routine (189-191). Such devices consist of a laser unit which is mounted to the CT-gantry or to a movable arm along an L-shaped rail (Figure 12).

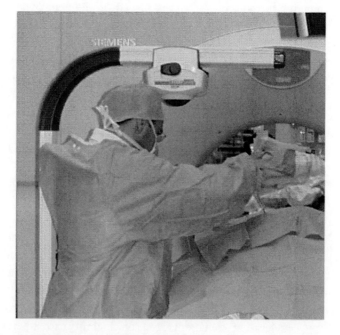

Figure 12. Laser guidance device SIMPLY-CT.

CT-Guided Radiofrequency Ablation of Liver Tumors

The device is independent of the scanner and software. The angles of the planned trajectory are manually entered into the operator panel and a laser beam is projected onto the patient, indicating entry and angulations of the planned trajectory. A comparative phantom analysis of freehand and laser-guided needle passes at varying single and double angles showed significant improved results for the laser-guidance with mean error of the laser guidance of 5.0 +/- 0.4 mm vs. standard freehand technique of 10.6 +/- 0.8 mm (192) (see Table 4). 93% of the laser-guided punctures and only 56% of the freehand punctures were within 1cm of the intended target (192). Puncture errors increase in both techniques with larger angles or double-angled approaches but the increase in errors is lower for the laser-guidance (192). In a clinical multicenter study a mean of 1.1 needle passes were required to reach the target and in 85% of patients the target was reached at the first attempt (189). Such results are hardly achieved with conventional freehand techniques.

Table 4. Targeting errors of CT-guided punctures

	Puncture technique	CT (slice thickness)	Error type	Mean +/- SD	Range	in/ex-vivo
Pereles et al. Acad Radiol 1998 (192)	Conventional guidance (single puncture)	n/a	Total Error	10,6 +/- 0,8 mm	n/a	Ex-vivo (phantom)
	Laser guidance		Total Error	5,0 +/- 0,4 mm	n/a	
Meyer et al. Invest Radiol 2001 (193)	Puncture guide	n/a	Angular Error (axial plane)	2,1° +/- 1,4°	0,2° - 4,6°	In-vivo (Patients)
			Angular Error (sagittal plane)	2,3° +/- 1,2°	0,4° - 4,0°	
Magnusson et al. Acta Radiol 2005 (194)	Puncture guide plus laser	n/a	Angular Error	2,4° +/- 2,4°	0° - 8°	In-vivo (Patients)
Crocetti et al. Invest Radiol 2008 (188)	Electromagnetic US-navigation	0,6 mm	Lateral Error (cytologic needle)	1,9 +/- 0,7 mm	0,8 – 3 mm	Ex-vivo (calf liver)
			Lateral Error (RF needle)	3,9 +/- 0,7 mm	2,9 – 5,1 mm	
Das et al. Radiology 2006 (231)	Optical navigation free-hand	1,5 mm	Total Error	3,5 +/- xx mm	2,7 – 4,2 mm	Ex-vivo (phantom)
Meier-Hein et al. Med Phys 2008 (212)	Optical navigation free-hand	1 mm	Total Error	2,6 +/- 1,7 mm	0,6 – 3,9 mm	In-vivo (pig)
Stoffer et al. Rofo 2009 (245)	Optical navigation stereotactic aiming device	1 mm	Total Error	1,94 +/- 0,91 mm	0,0 – 4,79 mm	Ex-vivo (phantom)
			Lateral Error	1,64 +/- 0,92 mm	0,0 – 4,75 mm	
		3 mm	Total Error	2,2 +/- 1,1 mm	0,6 – 5,5 mm	
			Lateral Error	1,8 +/- 1,2 mm	0,1 – 5,0 mm	

Table 4. (Continued)

Widmann et al. Minm Invasive Ther Allied Technol 2011 (205)	Optical navigation stereotactic aiming device	3 mm	Lateral Error	3,59 +/- 2,51 mm	0,0 – 14 mm	In-vivo (Patients)
			Angular Error	1,28° +/- 1,19°	0,0° - 7,99°	
Stoffer et al. Rofo 2009 (245)	Medical robot	1 mm	Total Error	1,69 +/- 0,77 mm	0,53 – 3,25 mm	Ex-vivo (phantom)
			Lateral Error	1,42 +/- 0,78 mm	0,18 – 3,07 mm	
		3 mm	Total Error	1,91 +/- 0,67 mm	0,95 – 3,87 mm	
			Lateral Error	1,6 +/- 0,73 mm	0,16 – 3,73 mm	Ex-vivo (phantom)
Kettenbach et al. Invest Radiol 2005 (252)	Medical robot	9 mm	Lateral Error (axial plane)	1.2 +/- 0.9 mm	0.0 – 2.5 mm	Ex-vivo (phantom)
			Lateral Error (sagittal plane)	0.6 +/- 0.4 mm	0.0 – 1.1 mm	

To further improve handling and puncture accuracy, *puncture guides* consisting of a base plate with a hemisphere and a tubular needle guide were developed (193-194). The puncture needle can rotate at the rotational center of the hemisphere on the base plate, which corresponds to the needle entry and the required angulations can be adjusted on the hemisphere. When angulations were adjusted using a scale for angulations on the axial plane (according to the angulations of the planned puncture path) and in the sagittal plane (according to the gantry angle), offsets between the puncture needles and the planned path were 2.1° +/- 1.4° (range 0.2° - 4.6°) in a patient study (193). Similar deviations were found when using a locking ring for fixation of the device during laser-guidance, with errors of 2.4° +/- 2.4° (range 0-8°) (194) (see Table 4). Compared to unsupported free-hand needle advancement these guidance devices provide stable needle advancement and guidance during double angulated puncture paths. Drawback is the limited maximum trajectory angle (+/- 30°), which may -under certain circumstances- preclude an intervention (194). In addition, the device has to be attached to the skin before imaging.

Virtual Sonography

Virtual sonography allow for treatment of lesions based on pre-interventional CT (and/or eventual MR) using US-guidance. The key element of this technology is the coupling of the US-transducer with an optical or electromagnetic based tracking system (57, 195) (Figure 13).

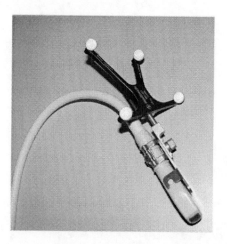

Figure 13. Virtual sonography using an optical tracked US-transducer.

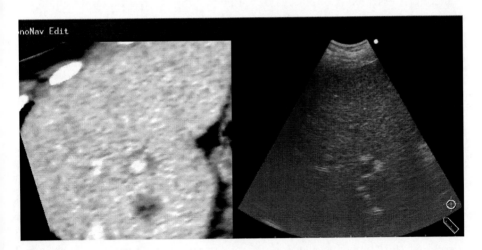

Figure 14. Reconstruction of 2-dimensional CT images (left) in identical orientation to the US images (right). Image of the first virtual sonography of the liver presented at RSNA 2002 by Bale et al.

2-dimensional CT images can be reconstructed identical in orientation to the US images (= real-time virtual sonography) (99, 196) (Figure 14). Thus, lesions which are even invisible in US may be treated by virtual sonography.

For the linkage of the real-time intraoperative US images to the corresponding multiplanar cross-sections of the preoperative CT, several techniques have been described. In *point-based registration*, skin markers can be defined in the image (manually or semi-automatically on the computer) and on the patient (with the probe of the navigation system) and the tracking system computes the geometrical transformation that best aligns these points (164, 178, 197). For high accuracy, 5-7 registration markers should be broadly distributed around the volume of interest and have to be clearly indicated on the image data and the patient, respectively (179, 198-200). In contrast, *image-based registration* may be performed by generation of an "orientation initialization" image by the tracked US transducer placed on the inferior end of the patient's sternum, parallel to a corresponding axial section of the CT (131). The registration is manually refined by matching characteristic vessel structures (e.g. umbilical portion of the right portal vein) on the virtual CT images and the B-mode US (131). Semi-automatic refinement can be performed by obtaining a subsequent series of US slices which is registered to the CT data using image transformation into probability images where the intensity values represent the probability of a voxel containing a vessel (178). Verification of correct image registration before puncture is essential. Corrections of the initial US-CT registration depending on the patient's position (e.g. left lateral position, elevated arm) or during different respiratory states may be necessary during the procedure to preserve acceptable registration accuracy. The most important prerequisite is respiratory triggering. The registration and the puncture should always be performed in the same respiratory state.

CT-based (0,6 mm slice thickness) electromagnetic US navigation with a 22G cytology needle allowed puncture of 1.5 mm targets in calf livers that were invisible in US with a mean lateral error of 1.9 +/- 0.7 mm (range 0.8 – 3.0 mm) (188). In the same study, placing expandable RFA probes at 1 cm from the center of the target with subsequent ablation, the mean lateral error was 3.9 +/- 0.7 mm (range 2.9 – 5.1 mm), the distance between the trocar and the target was 10.3 +/- 2.6 mm (range 6.3 – 14.3 mm) and the target was found in the center of the ablation zone in all cases (188). In comparison, MR-based optical US navigation permitted 100% puncture success of 6 mm targets in an abdominal phantom and showed targeting errors of 1-5.7 mm in an animal experiment (179).

CT-based US-navigated RFA provided a success rate of the first puncture in 90% of HCCs which were undetectable by conventional sonography (99). Real-time tracking of the electrode via tracking elements that are connected to the electrode allows for calculating and displaying the needle tip location and angulations and its predicted path with respect to the US transducer. Such a technology permits precise and fast targeting and can be used for out-of-plane approaches. As US navigation provides virtual information the verification of the confirmation of needle position after puncture and before RFA is important in this procedure in order to confirm needle insertion into the tumor and to reliably rule out perforations and other complications (99).

In HCCs which are poorly defined on B-mode US, US-navigated RFA can significantly improve technical success (in a single session in 92%, in two sessions in 8%), compared to B-mode US-guided RFA (in a single session in 72%, in two sessions in 24%, and in three sessions in 4%) (131).

Stereotactic RFA (SRFA)

The success of RFA is excellent for small lesions sized less than 3 cm; however, the results of large (diameter >3–5 cm) and irregularly shaped (non spherical) lesions as well as lesions located subcapsular or close to major vessels are unsatisfying and may argue for excluding such lesions from RFA-treatment (47, 79, 103, 124, 201-203). Reasons for technical failure may be poor visibility of the lesion and/or lesions borders during interventional imaging, difficulty of complex planning for multi-electrode ablations, imprecise electrode placement, insufficient ablation size, the heat sink effect due to vicinity to large vessels resulting, and insufficient application of energy (48, 79, 201).

To overcome the limitations of previous RFA techniques, stereotactic radiofrequency ablation (SRFA) has been implemented. SRFA combines CT imaging, computerized 3D planning of electrode positions and guided electrode placement at arbitrary angulations and orientations (19, 123, 175). The novel technology may substantially improve the technical possibilities of percutaneous tumor ablation.

PATIENT FIXATION AND RESPIRATORY MOTION CONTROL

Precise stereotactic placement of RF electrodes in the liver is only achievable when the imaged body region is a stationary volume unaffected by patient movements, arm position and respiration phase (57, 175, 180, 204-205). The patient has to remain exactly in the same position as in the precedent imaging procedure to ensure constant correspondence of imaged body regions. The motions of the intervention table must not influence the patient's stable position. Immobilization of the patient can be successfully achieved with vacuum cushion *patient fixation* systems (164, 204, 206-208). Such devices consist of a cushion which is filled with tiny Styrofoam balls (similar to a vacuum splint). When the vacuum pump is turned on, the air is evacuated resulting in a hardening of the cushion against the patient (204, 206) (Figure 15).

For accurate image-to-patient registration the images and the patient have to be matched in the same respiratory phase (131, 159, 204). Monitoring of the respiratory movement may be non-invasively obtained by using a reference marker or skin markers placed at the patient's skin. The markers are constantly detected by the tracking system during the intervention and enable a real-time update of the image-to-patient transformation (159, 180). Other techniques use a combination of 3D navigation and motion-triggered robotic assistance (197, 209). However, the accuracy of motion triggering is dependent on a consistent breathing pattern and cannot record internal motion of the liver. In contrast, invasive liver tracking may be performed by implanted tracked needles and a modified orientation-based registration algorithm, or by placement of an electromagnetic tracker wedged catheter into the hepatic vein (180, 210-212). Using these techniques, the target organ itself is tracked, but the invasiveness of the treatment increases.

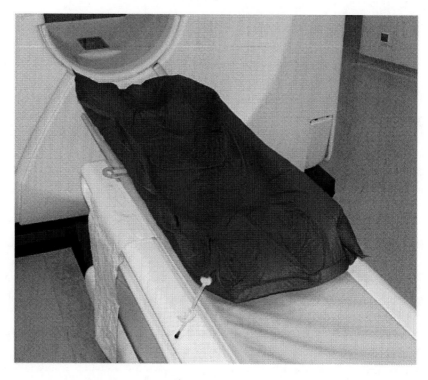

Figure 15. Vacuum cushion for patient fixation.

Research in elastic registration and tracking may help bridging the gap between the stiff snap-shots in cross-sectional imaging and the moving anatomical structures in the real patient (213-216). However, accurate elastic registration has still the drawback to be time consuming and thus it is not yet applicable in clinical routine navigation. In addition artificial virtual deformation of the liver may lead to unacceptable inaccuracies.

In practice, *respiratory motion compensation* can be successfully achieved when the interventional imaging, the registration procedure and the puncture are performed in maximal expiration. In critical cases with small or difficult targets and potential danger of puncture related complications such as laceration of vessels or treatment dependent collateral damage, excellent cooperation of the patient is required (9). However, such cooperation may not be warranted during uncomfortable patient positioning, pain or anxiety (9). Moreover, it is frequently difficult for patients with severe illness to hold their breath, even for a few seconds. In these cases, general anesthesia is required (175). In anaesthetised patients respiratory motion control can be successfully achieved by temporary disconnection of the endotracheal tube (ETT) (175, 204-205) (Figure 16).

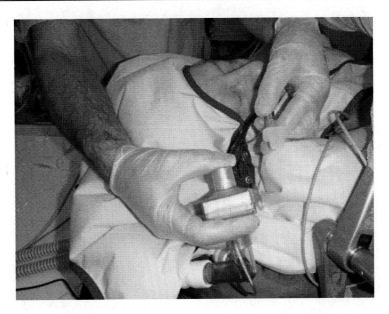

Figure 16. Temporary ETT disconnection under control of the anaesthetist in the intervention room.

During ETT disconnection, the paralysed patients end in a standardized end expiration state that is uninfluenced by pressures within the ventilation machine. The entire procedure is executed and controlled by the attending anaesthetist in the intervention room and monitored via live-video by the radiation technician and interventional radiologist. Temporary ETT disconnections are required during the CT scan, the electrode placement and control CTs. The temporary interruption of air supply is well tolerated by the patients and does not produce any noticed complications during or after anaesthesia (204). The overall error of respiratory motion control calculated using internal landmarks of the liver and external surface markers covering the area of the liver showed mean values of 1.69 ± 0.89 mm and a range of 0.44 – 4.02 mm (204).

NAVIGATION SYSTEMS

Frameless stereotactic navigation systems are already widely used in radiotherapy and various surgical procedures (neurosurgery, orthopedic surgery, ENT, craniomaxillofacial surgery). They represent a useful instrument for planning and precise transposition of the plan to the patient, thus permitting interventions whose success heavily depends on the accurate and reliable targeting of structures. Navigation systems are composed of a transportable workstation, a high-resolution display, a graphical user interface and several software applications, a position measuring system, and various probes or tracking adapters which can be mounted to surgical tools (175, 217). The guidance system or position measuring system (PMS) works similar to that of the global positioning system (GPS) in cars: Similar to the satellite, an optical or electromagnetic device detects tracking elements, which are mounted to a dynamic reference frame (DRF) on the patient, and to the surgical tools and calculates the position of the surgical tool in relation to the DRF.

Optical navigation systems are based on active emitting or passive reflecting light tracking elements which are mounted to a probe and recorded by a stereoscopic camera (123, 175) (Figure 17). They offer the advantage of a high accuracy for position recording in the range of 0.4 – 0.6 mm, convenient handling and easy sterilization (218).

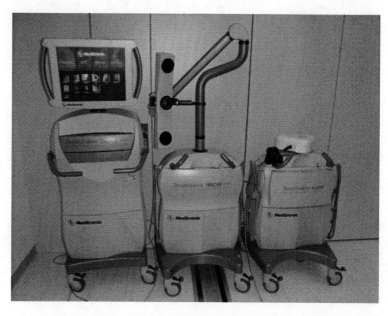

Figure 17. Navigation system with both, optical and electromagnetic tracking technology (Medtronic). Left – Workstation and high-resolution touch screen. Middle – Optical tracking provided by a stereoscopic camera. Right – Magnetic tracking provided by a magnetic field generator.

Disadvantages are the necessity of constant visual contact between camera-array, DRF and instruments and the potential susceptibility to interference through light reflexes on metallic surfaces in the operating environment (217, 219-220).

Electromagnetic navigation systems do not require visual contact between instrument and sensor system (57, 180, 210, 221-223) (Figure 17). An electromagnetic field generator produces a low electromagnetic field that enables tracking of the position and orientation of sensor coils. A weak current is induced in the sensor coil within the interventional device, and this current strength is dependent on location (131, 180, 217). Electromagnetic systems may reach comparable accuracy to optical systems but are sensitive to external magnetic fields and metal objects leading to incorrect position sensing of up to 4 mm (224-229). They are a relative contraindication for patients with pacemakers and cochlear implants (230).

3D TREATMENT PLANNING

The planning of electrode positions is based on the interventional CT. Additionally, multi modality fusion of CT, MRI, and PET or SPECT may be used for treatment planning (175, 213).

3D planning software on navigation systems allows for trajectory planning on different representations of the reformatted data, exploiting volume- and surface-rendering methods as well as advanced image processing with image segmentation and other medical image computing methods (19, 123, 175). Dedicated targeting graphics show the position of the tip or the 3D representation of the puncture device in relation to the predefined target / trajectory. Such graphics may consist of simple crosshair projections of the tip (in axial, sagittal and coronal plane or in 3D), "trajectory views" (longitudinal cuts along the guided trajectory), "probe's eye view" (perpendicular cuts to the guided trajectory), "guidance view" (showing distances off plan and angle of deviation of the tracked surgical tool from the surgical path), and "3D view" (3D reconstructions of puncture device, planned trajectory and target) (123) (Figure 18). Virtual flights along the planned trajectory may allow for visualization of vital structures close to the path or other obstacles already during the planning step, thereby minimizing the risk of collateral damage. Projection of virtual treatment zones obtained by various electrodes, displayed with predefined shapes and sizes based on mathematical ablation models may facilitate and improve treatment planning (57).

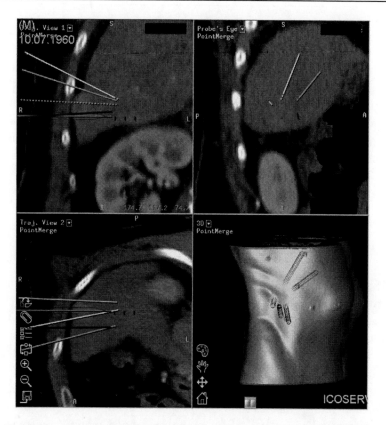

Figure 18. 3D planning for SRFA. HCC sized 4 cm, subcapsular in Segment VI, 5 coaxial needles/5 electrode positions (3 cm active extension). Upper left and Lower right – Trajectory views. Upper right – Probe's eye view. Lower right – 3D view.

IMAGE-TO-PATIENT REGISTRATION

Image-to-patient registration is usually performed using *paired-point registration* based on attachable skin markers (57, 175) (Figure 19). The placement of the registration markers is easy and quick and the entire registration procedure including CT imaging and data transfer may take approximately 10-15 minutes, (231). Alternatively, invasive marker needles may be placed in the liver to allow referencing the target organ itself (212, 232). Usually the markers have to be defined on the image date and consecutively indicated with the probe of the navigation system. In contrast, actively tracked markers paired with automatic segmentation on the pre-procedural scan may significantly reduce registration time (233).

CT-Guided Radiofrequency Ablation of Liver Tumors

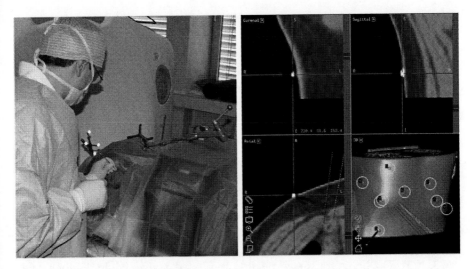

Figure 19. Paired-point registration using skin fiducial markers. Left - Touching fiducial markers on the patient with the probe of the navigation system. Right – Indicated surface markers on the navigation software in coronal, sagital, axial and 3D view.

In *modality based registration*, the positions of the CT gantry relative to the patient are tracked by the navigation system and the transformation from image to patient space is automatically calculated (208, 234-236). Automated registration technology is independent from manual definition of registration markers and may facilitate application (208, 235-236).

After registration, the navigation accuracy should be checked by touching uniquely identifiable points on the patient and comparing real and visualized position.

STEREOTACTIC TARGETING

During *3D-navigated stereotactic puncture* the "guidance view" and the "3D view" with data on distances off plan and angle of deviation are most helpful for trajectory alignment. In the guidance view a perpendicular projection of the trajectory is displayed and the actual tip and the end of the instrument are projected onto the trajectory in real-time (123, 175, 212).

Optical free-hand navigated CT-based (1.5 mm slice thickness) in-vitro targeting in a phantom provided a total puncture error of 3.5 mm (range 2.7 to 4.2 mm) and 100% success in first attempt to target simulated liver lesions sized in the range of 5-15 mm (231). Optical free-hand navigated CT-based (1 mm slice thickness) in-vivo targeting of artificial liver lesion in the swine using two invasive registration needles for registration showed total puncture errors of 2.6 +/- 1.7 mm (range 0.6 – 3.9 mm) (212) (see Table 4). With electromagnetic CT-based navigation, total errors during abdominal phantom punctures of about 4 mm have been reported (237).

Stereotactic Aiming Devices

Free-hand guidance may be hampered by complex hand-eye coordination, drift, and natural tremor. It can be difficult to move a tracked surgical tool in precise intervals relative to a target, exactly following the predefined trajectory while maintaining the aim on the target. In contrast, stereotactic aiming devices can be used for rigid stereotactic guidance of the probe advancement to the target (123, 175). The first retractors or flexible arm-based devices could rigidly hold the guidance probe for trajectory alignment in various positions (238-239). A drawback of such devices is that adjustment of the probe of the navigation system to the planned path is cumbersome. Next generation aiming devices consist of adjustable mechanical arms with up to 6 degrees of freedom which are connected to the intervention table and have guidance facilities at the head.

Easytaxis

The EasyTaxis aiming device (Philips Medical Systems Inc.) contains a spherical alignment body (trapped ball) at the head, that rotates freely in a lockable bearing (240-244). For trajectory alignment, the navigation probe is placed in a block with an incomplete inner bore that places the probe tip at the geometric center of the trapped ball. First, the tip of the navigation probe is placed at the virtual elongated trajectory of the planned path and the three joints of the mechanical arm are simultaneously locked in this position with one screw. Second, the navigation probe is rotated until it is aligned with the planned trajectory and the trapped ball is secured by a second screw. The distance from the tip of the navigation probe to the target is calculated to provide the correct puncture depth. The locked ball contains a central channel to accept tubes with varying inner bores of 2 – 5.25 mm calibre for the guidance of different instruments (243).

Vertek

The Vertek aiming device (Medtronic Inc., Louisville, USA) contains two independent pivot joints which rotate around two centers of rotation at the tip of the introduced navigation probe (241, 245-249) (Figure 20). The distance from the tip of the navigation probe is calculated to provide the correct targeting length. For guidance of various instruments, tubes with different inner bores have to be introduced in the head of the Vertek.

Atlas

The Atlas (Medical Intelligence, Schwabmünchen, Germany) is similar to the Vertek. In contrast, Atlas contains brackets with a freely adjustable concentric aperture which allows the use of tools with different calibres without needing to introduce dedicated tubes (205, 241, 245, 247-248).

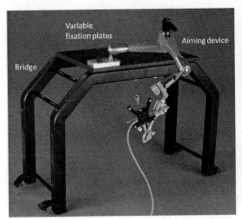 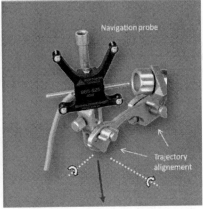

Figure 20. Vertek aiming device. Left – the aiming device is mounted to the bridge which can be connected to the intervention table. Right – Detail of the distal extension which allows for adjustments of angulations simplified by two pivot joints.

The navigation probe has to be removed once the trajectory has been aligned and the calculated depth from the aiming device to the target is marked on the electrode (19, 123, 175) (Figure 21). In contrast, if the electrode is provided with tracking elements (tracked electrode), the introduction of the electrode is continuously tracked with the assurance of exact alignment. One can both define his trajectory and depth within the software and monitor instrument location on-screen in real time.

In a phantom study, optical navigated stereotactic CT-guided (3 mm slice thickness) surface marker paired-point registration based punctures showed total targeting errors of 2.2 ± 1.1 mm (range $0.6 - 5.5$ mm) and lateral errors of 1.8 ± 1.2 mm (range $0.1 - 5.0$ mm) (245) (see Table 4).

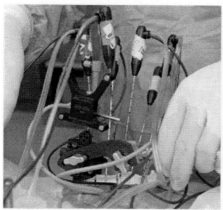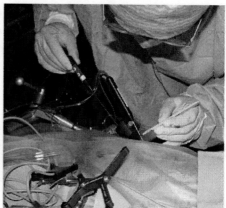

Figure 21. Stereotactic aiming device guided RF electrode placement. Left – Navigated adjustment of the aiming device. Right – RF electrode placement rigidly guided by the aiming device.

In a clinical study including 20 patients, the mean lateral error for optical navigated stereotactic CT-guided (3 mm slice thickness) stereotactic punctures was 2.59 ± 1.55 mm (range 0.2 – 9 mm) at the needle entry, 3.59 ± 2.51 mm (range 0.0 – 14 mm) at the needle tip, and the mean angular error was 1.28° ± 1.19° (range 0.0° – 7.99°) (205) (see Table 4). The mean longitudinal error at the needle tip was -7.4 ± 6.18 mm (range -41 – +3 mm) (205). Negative longitudinal errors reflected needle positions that were shorter than the corresponding plan, positive longitudinal errors reflected needle positions that were longer. Time efforts for the registration procedure including placement of registration markers, contrast enhanced CT-scan during ETT disconnection, data transfer to the navigation system, marker definition on the navigation software and marker indication with the navigation probe were approximately 10-15 minutes (205). The planning of one trajectory depends on the difficulty of the access route and needs approximately 2-5 minutes (205). For trajectory alignment with the stereotactic aiming device and placement of a single needle during temporary ETT disconnection, approximately 1-2 minutes are needed (205).

Medical Robots

Robots for image-guided interventions consist of computer-controlled mechanical arms with 6 to 7 degrees of freedom (250). The robot is either connected to a mobile platform or to the intervention table (Figure 22). For tracking of the robotic movements in space, optical tracking technology may be used (250-252). The tracking elements are mounted to the robotic arm and position recording is the same as in 3D-navigation. Alternatively, mechanical based tracking can be provided by internal sensors within the robotic arm. Mechanical based position recording is not influenced by imperfections in position sensing (e.g. jitter, geometrical distortions, etc.), which can be up to 20-40% of total localization error in optical tracking, or up to 50% in electromagnetic tracking (195, 225).

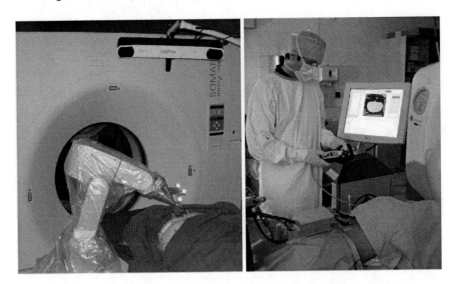

Figure 22. Medical robots for interventional radiology. Left – Full automated robotic arm for trajectory alignment. Right – Remote controlled miniature robot for trajectory alignment.

As a prerequisite for robotic interventions, a registration procedure similar to that of 3D-navigation is required. In contrast to flexible robots using registration markers, table-fixed robotic systems may be linked to the scanner machine and may provide automated, modality-based registration of the robot and use the coordinates of the image data for navigation (164, 245). Robots are expected to be more accurate and more reliable than a human being. They are immune to infection or radiation and can be automatically programmed for documentation, evaluation and training protocols. Robots can work as part of an interactive system with passive and active assistance. Passive robotic systems may be used for automated aiming of the planned insertion path at the center of a target. The subsequent advancement of the needle into the tumor is performed manually by the interventionalist using a coaxial technique (252). In contrast active robotics systems may automatically perform the entire targeting procedure, monitored by the interventionalist (250-251).

CT-guided (9 mm slice thickness) robot-assisted targeting of peas embedded within a gel phantom provided 1.2 +/- 0.9 mm (range 0.0 – 2.5 mm) and 0.6 +/- 0.4 mm (range 0.0 – 1.1 mm) in the axial and sagittal plane, respectively (252) (see Table 4). Using an active robot system which is connected to the CT-table, in-vitro puncture based on 1-, and 3 mm CT scans and automated modality-based registration showed a total puncture error of 1.7 +/- 0.8 mm (range 0.5 – 3.3 mm), and 1.9 +/- 0.7 mm (range 1.0 – 3.9 mm), respectively (245) (see Table 4). Although the robot was more accurate than stereotaxy with an aiming device, significant differences could not be observed (245).

In robotic targeting, several issues influence accuracy: inappropriate calibration of the robotic components, small movements of the robotic arm due to minor mechanical instabilities or bending when fully extended, and deflections of the targeting device by inhomogeneous tissue structures during puncture (252). Many systems still have improper planning tools and need relatively long time for preparation and set-up (253). In a comparative study, the robotic system needed approx. 25 min. for one puncture set-up (including the time needed for image acquisition, autocalibration, registration, data transfer and planning of a single puncture) vs. 15 min for the navigation system (including the time for image acquisition, data transfer, camera alignment, tool calibration, and planning of a single puncture), and approx. 5 min. vs. 2.5 min for a single needle insertion (245).

Monitoring and Treatment Evaluation

Verification of the needle position after puncture and before RFA is important in order to confirm needle placement into the tumor and to reliably rule out perforations and other complications (99). The control CT is usually performed without contrast and with the same slice thickness as for the planning CT. The fusion of the control-images to the planning data allows for an immediate check of the electrode position in relation to the plan (19, 123, 175) (Figure 23). When placement of more than three RF electrodes is required, use of coaxial needles is advised (19, 123). After verification of the correct position, the RF electrodes may be inserted via the coaxial needles and placed tip to tip. Afterwards the shorter coaxial needles need to be retracted in order to uncover the active electrode exposure. Thus, repeat imaging for electrode positioning control may not be required.

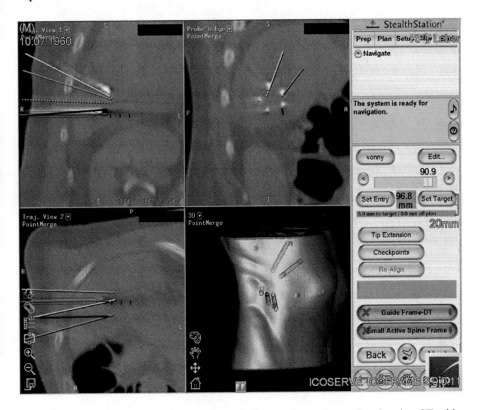

Figure 23. Fusion of the native control CT with the needles in situ to the planning CT with the stored plans. Note the precise position almost exactly aligned with the plan. Right column – the measurements indicate that the needle needs to be advanced 5.9 mm to be exactly at the planned position.

Real-time monitoring of the ablation using CT is not feasible due to unjustifiable radiation exposition. After RFA, the ablation zone is immediately evaluated in a contrast enhanced control CT with the electrodes in situ or after needle retraction to rule out puncture related complications and collateral ablative damage. After RFA, superposition of the post-ablation images to the planning data using image fusion provides an optimal comparison of the obtained ablation necrosis with the initial tumor by blending from one image to the other, rather than comparing the images mentally side-by-side (19, 57, 123, 175, 254) (Figure 24).

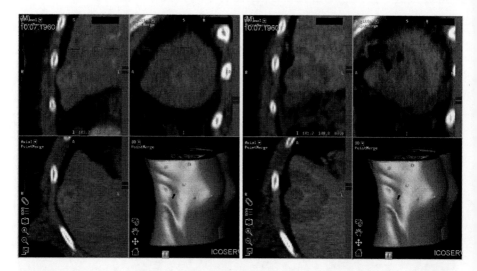

Figure 24. Image fusion of enhanced control CT immediately after RFA with the planning CT. Left – Blend setting 0, planning CT showing the tumor. Right – Blend setting 100, control CT showing the ablation. Note the large safety margin included in the hypodense ablation area with respect of the initial hyperdense tumor.

On unenhanced CT immediately after treatment, the RF lesion has approximately 22 Houndsfield units (HU) lower values compared to the surrounding liver (lower than liver) (133). Unenhanced CT correlates better to the pathologic size as compared to contrast-enhanced CT, but contrast-enhanced CT best correlates with lesion shape (133). Contrast-enhanced CT shows a circumscribed non-enhancing ablation region surrounded by a reactive rim enhancement (3, 255-256). The ring like enhancement around the ablation zone represents benign reactive hyperemia. Central areas of high attenuation represent greater cellular disruption (e.g. protein denaturation) and may be combined with tiny air bubbles (257). One has to regard that contrast-enhanced CT slightly overestimates the size due to areas of ischemia surrounding the RF lesion (133). As probably every image modality, CT imaging tends to overestimate the success of RFA when compared to the histopatholgic findings (149). Differences of complete histologic response rate after RFA vs. radiologic response rate of 7-15% have been reported (15).

Additional CT is absolutely necessary in patients with ongoing pain or suspicious complications such as infection or visceral perforation (96, 257).

Follow-up Imaging

The following time points for control CTs after RFA may be used (94):

- 1 month: control for residual tumor tissue (technique effectiveness)
- 3, 6, 9, and 12 months and at 6-month intervals thereafter for the next 3 years: control for new tumor tissue (local recurrence, distant intrahepatic recurrence, or extrahepatic disease)

The following standard protocol may be recommended:

- 5 mm helical native scan of the liver
- i.v. 90-120 ml Iodixanol 320 mg J/mg, 3ml/sec:

  - 3 mm contrast enhanced scan of the liver in the arterial phase
  - 3 mm (5 mm) contrast enhanced scan of the liver (abdomen) in the portal phase
  - 3 mm contrast enhanced scan of the liver in the late phase.

Arterial, portal and late phase are used for HCC and intrahepatic cholangiocellular carcinoma. Arterial and portal phase are used in neuroendocrine tumours. For all other tumor entities and metastases, portal phase scans may be sufficient.

CT Radiographic Signs at Follow-up after RFA

Void of contrast enhancement of a previously enhancing tumor is a reliable predictor of tissue necrosis. Demonstration of a sharp coagulation margin is important, because diffuse margins were significantly associated with local recurrence (258). Coagulation diameters that are smaller than the preoperative tumor diameter in the one month follow-up CT-scans are associated with local tumor progression (259). 3D volumetric analysis compared with conventional morphologic criteria could not provide significant advantages in early detection of local tumor progression (259).

Within one month it may be difficult to identify residual tumor tissue because of the peripheral enhancement around the ablated area (257) (Figure 25).

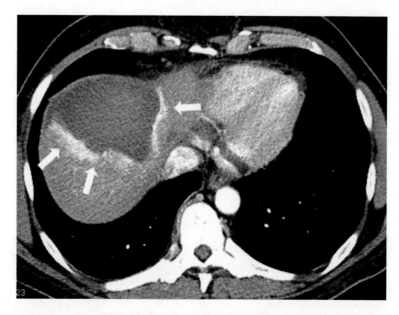

Figure 25. Reactive peripheral hypervascularization at contrast-enhanced CT 1 month after RFA. Note the strong hypervascular rim (white arrows) around the ablation zone.

The typical hypervascular rim disappears approximately one to three months after treatment and hypervascularized residual tumor tissue (such as HCC) can be differentiated from the RFA induced peripheral hypervascularity (260). Early differentiation between hypovascular metastastic lesions from avascular RFA induced necrosis may difficult and has to be suspected by any distortion in the smooth interface of the ablation zone (257, 261).

Usually, the size of the RFA necrosis shrinks during the time, and shrinkage at all borders is a very good indicator for successful treatment (181, 257) (Figure 26).

Because tumor tissue is devitalized (including a safety margin of healthy tissue) and not removed surgically, the World Health Organization (WHO) or Response Evaluation Criteria in Solid Tumors (RECIST) criteria, which are dependent on the size measurement of target lesions are insufficient to describe treatment success of RFA (262-264). Modified criteria that include the enhancement during contrast imaging should be recommended (263). More recently, (semi)automated evaluation of liver lesions treated by RFA, including volumetric assessment and HU measures before and after RFA may facilitate and improve treatment evaluation (182-183, 265). Consequently, every new increase in size and peripheral (nodal) hypervascularization is strongly suspicious for local recurrence (Figure 27).

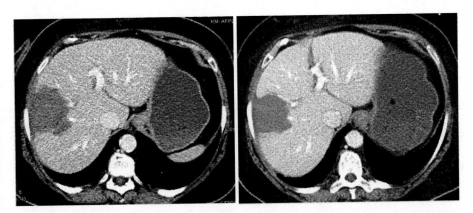

Figure 26. Shrinkage of the size in all borders of the RFA necrosis during time. Left – Contrast-enhanced CT 1 month after RFA. Right – Contrast-enhanced CT 12 months after RFA.

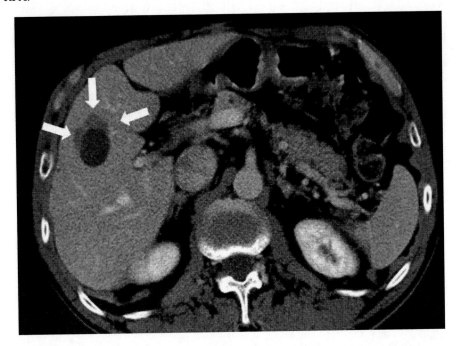

Figure 27. Local recurrence after RFA. Note the irregular hypovascular lesion (white arrows) around the ventral border of the dark ablation necrosis in the contrast-enhanced CT 2 years after RFA.

PET-CT may increase the detection rate for residual tumor and is superior to functional imaging alone (152). A sensitivity of 65% and an accuracy of 68% have been reported for detection of residual tumor with PET-CT vs. 44% and 47%, respectively for CT alone using the standard of reference based on clinical and radiologic follow-up (266). In a clinical study including sixteen patients with 25 18-FDG (fluor deoxy glucose) positive colorectal liver metastases treated with RFA, the accuracy and sensitivity for detection of local tumor progression was 86% and 76% for PET alone, 91% and 83% for PET-CT and 92% and 75% for MR, respectively (152). 18-FDG-PET immediately after RFA shows no increase in uptake, whereas elevated contrast enhancement is noted in the periphery of the ablation necrosis on all morphologic image modalities (261). However, between day 3 up to 6 months after RFA, regenerative tissue changes in the periphery of the ablation necrosis induce increased 18-FDG uptake which may superimpose on small areas of residual tumor and produce false negative results (261, 266). As a consequence, PET or PET-CT has to be performed either immediately or 6 months after RFA (261). One has to regard that PET has a limited spatial resolution of approximately 4 – 6 mm and sensitivity decreases dramatically in lesions less than 1 cm, so very small residual tumor may be missed (266). Further, obesity reduces PET image quality and (neo-) adjuvant chemotherapy decreases FDG-uptake (267-268). PET/SPECT imaging is only useful for tumors with preinterventional positive tracer uptake (152). Compared to morphologic imaging modalities such as US, CEUS or CT, PET/SPECT is less available and limited to larger clinical centers. Combined PET/SPECT-CT scanner further increase overall radiation exposure as required for a PET/SPECT or CT alone, which limits its use for routine sequential follow-up imaging.

CONCLUSION

In recent years, percutaneous RFA has emerged as an attractive local treatment of primary or secondary liver malignancies. Goal is to successfully ablate the tumor and a sufficient intentional margin of healthy tissue to provide maximum local tumor control similar to surgical resection. To achieve this goal, overlapping ablations have to be precisely planned and executed. Newer technology including CT-guided 3D-navigated stereotaxy may substantially increase the technical possibilities and effectiveness of RFA, by integration of 3D-imaging, computerized planning and stereotactic guided electrode placement. Due to its minimal invasiveness with low morbidity and mortality rates and short hospital stays RFA might become an attractive alternative to the standard surgical approach.

REFERENCES

[1] Gazelle GS, Goldberg SN, Solbiati L, Livraghi T. *Tumor ablation with radio-frequency energy*. Radiology. 2000 Dec;217(3):633-46.

[2] Goldberg SN, Gazelle GS, Mueller PR. *Thermal ablation therapy for focal malignancy: a unified approach to underlying principles, techniques, and diagnostic imaging guidance*. Ajr. 2000 Feb;174(2):323-31.

[3] Rhim H, Goldberg SN, Dodd GD, 3rd, Solbiati L, Lim HK, Tonolini M, et al. *Essential techniques for successful radio-frequency thermal ablation of malignant hepatic tumors*. Radiographics. 2001 Oct;21 Spec No:S17-35; discussion S6-9.

[4] Dupuy DE, Goldberg SN. *Image-guided radiofrequency tumor ablation: challenges and opportunities--part II*. J Vasc Interv Radiol. 2001 Oct;12(10):1135-48.

[5] Choti MA, Sitzmann JV, Tiburi MF, Sumetchotimetha W, Rangsin R, Schulick RD, et al. *Trends in long-term survival following liver resection for hepatic colorectal metastases*. Annals of surgery. 2002 Jun;235(6):759-66.

[6] Robertson DJ, Stukel TA, Gottlieb DJ, Sutherland JM, Fisher ES. *Survival after hepatic resection of colorectal cancer metastases: a national experience*. Cancer. 2009 Feb 15;115(4):752-9.

[7] Virani S, Michaelson JS, Hutter MM, Lancaster RT, Warshaw AL, Henderson WG, et al. *Morbidity and mortality after liver resection: results of the patient safety in surgery study*. J Am Coll Surg. 2007 Jun;204(6):1284-92.

[8] Mulier S, Mulier P, Ni Y, Miao Y, Dupas B, Marchal G, et al. *Complications of radiofrequency coagulation of liver tumours*. The British journal of surgery. 2002 Oct;89(10):1206-22.

[9] Livraghi T, Solbiati L, Meloni MF, Gazelle GS, Halpern EF, Goldberg SN. *Treatment of focal liver tumors with percutaneous radio-frequency ablation: complications encountered in a multicenter study*. Radiology. 2003 Feb;226(2):441-51.

[10] Curley SA, Marra P, Beaty K, Ellis LM, Vauthey JN, Abdalla EK, et al. *Early and late complications after radiofrequency ablation of malignant liver tumors in 608 patients*. Annals of surgery. 2004 Apr;239(4):450-8.

56   Gerlig Widmann and Reto Bale

[11] Lau WY, Lai EC. *The current role of radiofrequency ablation in the management of hepatocellular carcinoma: a systematic review.* Annals of surgery. 2009 Jan;249(1):20-5.

[12] Sutherland LM, Williams JA, Padbury RT, Gotley DC, Stokes B, Maddern GJ. *Radiofrequency ablation of liver tumors: a systematic review.* Arch Surg. 2006 Feb;141(2):181-90.

[13] Yao FY, Hirose R, LaBerge JM, Davern TJ, 3rd, Bass NM, Kerlan RK, Jr., et al. *A prospective study on downstaging of hepatocellular carcinoma prior to liver transplantation.* Liver Transpl. 2005 Dec;11(12):1505-14.

[14] Yao FY, Kinkhabwala M, LaBerge JM, Bass NM, Brown R, Jr., Kerlan R, et al. *The impact of pre-operative loco-regional therapy on outcome after liver transplantation for hepatocellular carcinoma.* Am J Transplant. 2005 Apr;5(4 Pt 1):795-804.

[15] Mazzaferro V, Battiston C, Perrone S, Pulvirenti A, Regalia E, Romito R, et al. *Radiofrequency ablation of small hepatocellular carcinoma in cirrhotic patients awaiting liver transplantation: a prospective study.* Annals of surgery. 2004 Nov;240(5):900-9.

[16] Solbiati L, Livraghi T, Goldberg SN, Ierace T, Meloni F, Dellanoce M, et al. *Percutaneous radio-frequency ablation of hepatic metastases from colorectal cancer: long-term results in 117 patients.* Radiology. 2001 Oct;221(1):159-66.

[17] Livraghi T, Goldberg SN, Solbiati L, Meloni F, Ierace T, Gazelle GS. *Percutaneous radio-frequency ablation of liver metastases from breast cancer: initial experience in 24 patients.* Radiology. 2001 Jul;220(1):145-9.

[18] Livraghi T, Solbiati L, Meloni F, Ierace T, Goldberg SN, Gazelle GS. *Percutaneous radiofrequency ablation of liver metastases in potential candidates for resection: the "test-of-time approach".* Cancer. 2003 Jun 15;97(12):3027-35.

[19] Bale R, Widmann G, Haidu M. *Stereotactic Radiofrequency Ablation.* Cardiovascular and interventional radiology. 2010 Aug 24.

[20] Carrafiello G, Lagana D, Cotta E, Mangini M, Fontana F, Bandiera F, et al. *Radiofrequency ablation of intrahepatic cholangiocarcinoma: preliminary experience.* Cardiovascular and interventional radiology. 2010 Aug;33(4):835-9.

[21] Lin SM, Lin CJ, Lin CC, Hsu CW, Chen YC. *Radiofrequency ablation improves prognosis compared with ethanol injection for hepatocellular carcinoma < or =4 cm.* Gastroenterology. 2004 Dec;127(6):1714-23.

[22] Shiina S, Teratani T, Obi S, Sato S, Tateishi R, Fujishima T, et al. *A randomized controlled trial of radiofrequency ablation with ethanol*

injection for small hepatocellular carcinoma. Gastroenterology. 2005 Jul;129(1):122-30.

[23] Lin SM, Lin CJ, Lin CC, Hsu CW, Chen YC. *Randomised controlled trial comparing percutaneous radiofrequency thermal ablation, percutaneous ethanol injection, and percutaneous acetic acid injection to treat hepatocellular carcinoma of 3 cm or less.* Gut. 2005 Aug;54(8):1151-6.

[24] Brunello F, Veltri A, Carucci P, Pagano E, Ciccone G, Moretto P, et al. *Radiofrequency ablation versus ethanol injection for early hepatocellular carcinoma: A randomized controlled trial.* Scand J Gastroenterol. 2008;43(6):727-35.

[25] Lencioni RA, Allgaier HP, Cioni D, Olschewski M, Deibert P, Crocetti L, et al. *Small hepatocellular carcinoma in cirrhosis: randomized comparison of radio-frequency thermal ablation versus percutaneous ethanol injection.* Radiology. 2003 Jul;228(1):235-40.

[26] Lencioni R, Cioni D, Crocetti L, Franchini C, Pina CD, Lera J, et al. *Early-stage hepatocellular carcinoma in patients with cirrhosis: long-term results of percutaneous image-guided radiofrequency ablation.* Radiology. 2005 Mar;234(3):961-7.

[27] Tateishi R, Shiina S, Teratani T, Obi S, Sato S, Koike Y, et al. *Percutaneous radiofrequency ablation for hepatocellular carcinoma. An analysis of 1000 cases.* Cancer. 2005 Mar 15;103(6):1201-9.

[28] Cabassa P, Donato F, Simeone F, Grazioli L, Romanini L. *Radiofrequency ablation of hepatocellular carcinoma: long-term experience with expandable needle electrodes.* Ajr. 2006 May;186(5 Suppl):S316-21.

[29] Choi D, Lim HK, Rhim H, Kim YS, Lee WJ, Paik SW, et al. *Percutaneous radiofrequency ablation for early-stage hepatocellular carcinoma as a first-line treatment: long-term results and prognostic factors in a large single-institution series.* European radiology. 2007 Mar;17(3):684-92.

[30] akahashi S, Kudo M, Chung H, Inoue T, Ishikawa E, Kitai S, et al. *Initial treatment response is essential to improve survival in patients with hepatocellular carcinoma who underwent curative radiofrequency ablation therapy.* Oncology. 2007;72 Suppl 1:98-103.

[31] Hiraoka A, Horiike N, Yamashita Y, Koizumi Y, Doi K, Yamamoto Y, et al. *Efficacy of radiofrequency ablation therapy compared to surgical resection in 164 patients in Japan with single hepatocellular carcinoma smaller than 3 cm, along with report of complications.* Hepato-gastroenterology. 2008 Nov-Dec;55(88):2171-4.

[32] Timmerman RD, Bizekis CS, Pass HI, Fong Y, Dupuy DE, Dawson LA, et al. *Local surgical, ablative, and radiation treatment of metastases.* CA Cancer J Clin. 2009 May-Jun;59(3):145-70.

[33] Ahmad A, Chen SL, Kavanagh MA, Allegra DP, Bilchik AJ. *Radiofrequency ablation of hepatic metastases from colorectal cancer: are newer generation probes better?* Am Surg. 2006 Oct;72(10):875-9.

[34] Lencioni R, Crocetti L, Cioni D, Della Pina C, Bartolozzi C. *Percutaneous radiofrequency ablation of hepatic colorectal metastases: technique, indications, results, and new promises.* Investigative radiology. 2004 Nov;39(11):689-97.

[35] Gillams AR, Lees WR. *Radio-frequency ablation of colorectal liver metastases in 167 patients.* European radiology. 2004 Dec;14(12):2261-7.

[36] Machi J, Oishi AJ, Sumida K, Sakamoto K, Furumoto NL, Oishi RH, et al. *Long-term outcome of radiofrequency ablation for unresectable liver metastases from colorectal cancer: evaluation of prognostic factors and effectiveness in first- and second-line management.* Cancer J. 2006 Jul-Aug;12(4):318-26.

[37] Veltri A, Sacchetto P, Tosetti I, Pagano E, Fava C, Gandini G. *Radiofrequency ablation of colorectal liver metastases: small size favorably predicts technique effectiveness and survival.* Cardiovascular and interventional radiology. 2008 Sep-Oct;31(5):948-56.

[38] Mulier S, Ni Y, Jamart J, Michel L, Marchal G, Ruers T. *Radiofrequency ablation versus resection for resectable colorectal liver metastases: time for a randomized trial?* Annals of surgical oncology. 2008 Jan;15(1):144-57.

[39] Goldberg SN, Solbiati L, Halpern EF, Gazelle GS. *Variables affecting proper system grounding for radiofrequency ablation in an animal model.* J Vasc Interv Radiol. 2000 Sep;11(8):1069-75.

[40] Goldberg SN, Gazelle GS, Solbiati L, Livraghi T, Tanabe KK, Hahn PF, et al. *Ablation of liver tumors using percutaneous RF therapy.* Ajr. 1998 Apr;170(4):1023-8.

[41] Goldberg SN, Gazelle GS, Halpern EF, Rittman WJ, Mueller PR, Rosenthal DI. *Radiofrequency tissue ablation: importance of local temperature along the electrode tip exposure in determining lesion shape and size.* Academic radiology. 1996 Mar;3(3):212-8.

[42] Goldberg SN, Gazelle GS, Dawson SL, Rittman WJ, Mueller PR, Rosenthal DI. *Tissue ablation with radiofrequency: effect of probe size, gauge, duration, and temperature on lesion volume.* Academic radiology. 1995 May;2(5):399-404.

CT-Guided Radiofrequency Ablation of Liver Tumors 59

[43] Patterson EJ, Scudamore CH, Owen DA, Nagy AG, Buczkowski AK. *Radiofrequency ablation of porcine liver in vivo: effects of blood flow and treatment time on lesion size.* Annals of surgery. 1998 Apr;227(4):559-65.

[44] Goldberg SN, Hahn PF, Halpern EF, Fogle RM, Gazelle GS. *Radio-frequency tissue ablation: effect of pharmacologic modulation of blood flow on coagulation diameter.* Radiology. 1998 Dec;209(3):761-7.

[45] Goldberg SN, Hahn PF, Tanabe KK, Mueller PR, Schima W, *Athanasoulis CA, et al. Percutaneous radiofrequency tissue ablation: does perfusion-mediated tissue cooling limit coagulation necrosis?* J Vasc Interv Radiol. 1998 Jan-Feb;9(1 Pt 1):101-11.

[46] Livraghi T, Goldberg SN, Lazzaroni S, Meloni F, Solbiati L, Gazelle GS. *Small hepatocellular carcinoma: treatment with radio-frequency ablation versus ethanol injection.* Radiology. 1999 Mar;210(3):655-61.

[47] Hori T, Nagata K, Hasuike S, Onaga M, Motoda M, Moriuchi A, et al. *Risk factors for the local recurrence of hepatocellular carcinoma after a single session of percutaneous radiofrequency ablation.* Journal of gastroenterology. 2003;38(10):977-81.

[48] Livraghi T, Goldberg SN, Lazzaroni S, Meloni F, Ierace T, Solbiati L, et al. *Hepatocellular carcinoma: radio-frequency ablation of medium and large lesions.* Radiology. 2000 Mar;214(3):761-8.

[49] Montgomery RS, Rahal A, Dodd GD, 3rd, Leyendecker JR, Hubbard LG. *Radiofrequency ablation of hepatic tumors: variability of lesion size using a single ablation device.* Ajr. 2004 Mar;182(3):657-61.

[50] Mulier S, Miao Y, Mulier P, Dupas B, Pereira P, de Baere T, et al. *Electrodes and multiple electrode systems for radiofrequency ablation: a proposal for updated terminology.* European radiology. 2005 Apr;15(4):798-808.

[51] Denys AL, De Baere T, Kuoch V, Dupas B, Chevallier P, Madoff DC, et al. *Radio-frequency tissue ablation of the liver: in vivo and ex vivo experiments with four different systems.* European radiology. 2003 Oct;13(10):2346-52.

[52] Mulier S, Ni Y, Miao Y, Rosiere A, Khoury A, Marchal G, et al. *Size and geometry of hepatic radiofrequency lesions.* Eur J Surg Oncol. 2003 Dec;29(10):867-78.

[53] Miao Y, Ni Y, Yu J, Zhang H, Baert A, Marchal G. *An ex vivo study on radiofrequency tissue ablation: increased lesion size by using an "expandable-wet" electrode.* European radiology. 2001;11(9):1841-7.

[54] Bruners P, Pfeffer J, Kazim RM, Gunther RW, Schmitz-Rode T, Mahnken AH. *A newly developed perfused umbrella electrode for radiofrequency*

ablation: an ex vivo evaluation study in bovine liver. Cardiovascular and interventional radiology. 2007 Sep-Oct;30(5):992-8.

[55] Pereira PL, Trubenbach J, Schenk M, Subke J, Kroeber S, Schaefer I, et al. *Radiofrequency ablation: in vivo comparison of four commercially available devices in pig livers.* Radiology. 2004 Aug;232(2):482-90.

[56] Martin RC, 2nd. *Intraoperative magnetic resonance imaging ablation of hepatic tumors.* Am J Surg. 2005 Apr;189(4):388-94.

[57] Wood BJ, Locklin JK, Viswanathan A, Kruecker J, Haemmerich D, Cebral J, et al. *Technologies for guidance of radiofrequency ablation in the multimodality interventional suite of the future.* J Vasc Interv Radiol. 2007 Jan;18(1 Pt 1):9-24.

[58] Mulier S, Ni Y, Frich L, Burdio F, Denys AL, De Wispelaere JF, et al. *Experimental and clinical radiofrequency ablation: proposal for standardized description of coagulation size and geometry.* Annals of surgical oncology. 2007 Apr;14(4):1381-96.

[59] Chen MH, Wei Y, Yan K, Gao W, Dai Y, Huo L, et al. *Treatment strategy to optimize radiofrequency ablation for liver malignancies.* J Vasc Interv Radiol. 2006 Apr;17(4):671-83.

[60] Sakuhara Y, Shimizu T, Abo D, Hasegawa Y, Kato F, Kodama Y, et al. *Influence of surgical staples on radiofrequency ablation using multitined expandable electrodes.* Cardiovascular and interventional radiology. 2007 Nov-Dec;30(6):1201-5.

[61] Lin SM, Lin CC, Chen WT, Chen YC, Hsu CW. *Radiofrequency ablation for hepatocellular carcinoma: a prospective comparison of four radiofrequency devices.* J Vasc Interv Radiol. 2007 Sep;18(9):1118-25.

[62] Head HW, Dodd GD, 3rd, Dalrymple NC, Prasad SR, El-Merhi FM, Freckleton MW, et al. *Percutaneous radiofrequency ablation of hepatic tumors against the diaphragm: frequency of diaphragmatic injury.* Radiology. 2007 Jun;243(3):877-84.

[63] McGahan JP, Gu WZ, Brock JM, Tesluk H, Jones CD. *Hepatic ablation using bipolar radiofrequency electrocautery.* Academic radiology. 1996 May;3(5):418-22.

[64] Goldberg SN, Gazelle GS, Solbiati L, Rittman WJ, Mueller PR. *Radiofrequency tissue ablation: increased lesion diameter with a perfusion electrode.* Academic radiology. 1996 Aug;3(8):636-44.

[65] Goldberg SN, Gazelle GS, Dawson SL, Rittman WJ, Mueller PR, Rosenthal DI. *Tissue ablation with radiofrequency using multiprobe arrays.* Academic radiology. 1995 Aug;2(8):670-4.

[66] Goldberg SN, Ahmed M, Gazelle GS, Kruskal JB, Huertas JC, Halpern EF, et al. *Radio-frequency thermal ablation with NaCl solution injection: effect of electrical conductivity on tissue heating and coagulation-phantom and porcine liver study.* Radiology. 2001 Apr;219(1):157-65.

[67] Ni Y, Miao Y, Mulier S, Yu J, Baert AL, Marchal G. *A novel "cooled-wet" electrode for radiofrequency ablation.* European radiology. 2000;10(5):852-4.

[68] Miao Y, Ni Y, Yu J, Marchal G. *A comparative study on validation of a novel cooled-wet electrode for radiofrequency liver ablation.* Investigative radiology. 2000 Jul;35(7):438-44.

[69] Lee JM, Han JK, Kim SH, Shin KS, Lee JY, Park HS, et al. *Comparison of wet radiofrequency ablation with dry radiofrequency ablation and radiofrequency ablation using hypertonic saline preinjection: ex vivo bovine liver.* Korean J Radiol. 2004 Oct-Dec;5(4):258-65.

[70] Livraghi T, Goldberg SN, Monti F, Bizzini A, Lazzaroni S, Meloni F, et al. *Saline-enhanced radio-frequency tissue ablation in the treatment of liver metastases.* Radiology. 1997 Jan;202(1):205-10.

[71] Lee JM, Han JK, Kim SH, Lee JY, Choi SH, Choi BI. *Hepatic bipolar radiofrequency ablation using perfused-cooled electrodes: a comparative study in the ex vivo bovine liver.* The British journal of radiology. 2004 Nov;77(923):944-9.

[72] Lee JM, Han JK, Kim SH, Lee JY, Shin KS, Han CJ, et al. *Optimization of wet radiofrequency ablation using a perfused-cooled electrode: a comparative study in ex vivo bovine livers.* Korean J Radiol. 2004 Oct-Dec;5(4):250-7.

[73] Lee JM, Han JK, Kim SH, Choi SH, An SK, Han CJ, et al. *Bipolar radiofrequency ablation using wet-cooled electrodes: an in vitro experimental study in bovine liver.* Ajr. 2005 Feb;184(2):391-7.

[74] Lee JM, Han JK, Kim SH, Lee JY, Kim DJ, Lee MW, et al. *Saline-enhanced hepatic radiofrequency ablation using a perfused-cooled electrode: comparison of dual probe bipolar mode with monopolar and single probe bipolar modes.* Korean J Radiol. 2004 Apr-Jun;5(2):121-7.

[75] Lee JM, Han JK, Kim SH, Sohn KL, Choi SH, Choi BI. *Bipolar radiofrequency ablation in ex vivo bovine liver with the open-perfused system versus the cooled-wet system.* European radiology. 2005 Apr;15(4):759-64.

[76] Lee JM, Kim SH, Han JK, Sohn KL, Choi BI. *Ex vivo experiment of saline-enhanced hepatic bipolar radiofrequency ablation with a perfused needle electrode: comparison with conventional monopolar and simultaneous*

62 Gerlig Widmann and Reto Bale

monopolar modes. Cardiovascular and interventional radiology. 2005 May-Jun;28(3):338-45.

[77] Lee JM, Han JK, Kim SH, Sohn KL, Lee KH, Ah SK, et al. *A comparative experimental study of the in-vitro efficiency of hypertonic saline-enhanced hepatic bipolar and monopolar radiofrequency ablation.* Korean J Radiol. 2003 Jul-Sep;4(3):163-9.

[78] Goldberg SN, Gazelle GS. *Radiofrequency tissue ablation: physical principles and techniques for increasing coagulation necrosis.* Hepato-gastroenterology. 2001 Mar-Apr;48(38):359-67.

[79] Rhim H, Lim HK, Kim YS, Choi D, Lee WJ. *Radiofrequency ablation of hepatic tumors: lessons learned from 3000 procedures.* Journal of gastroenterology and hepatology. 2008 Oct;23(10):1492-500.

[80] Goldberg SN, Solbiati L, Hahn PF, Cosman E, Conrad JE, Fogle R, et al. *Large-volume tissue ablation with radio frequency by using a clustered, internally cooled electrode technique: laboratory and clinical experience in liver metastases.* Radiology. 1998 Nov;209(2):371-9.

[81] Laeseke PF, Sampson LA, Haemmerich D, Brace CL, Fine JP, Frey TM, et al. Multiple-electrode radiofrequency ablation: simultaneous production of separate zones of coagulation in an in vivo porcine liver model. J Vasc Interv Radiol. 2005 Dec;16(12):1727-35.

[82] Lee JM, Han JK, Kim HC, Choi YH, Kim SH, Choi JY, et al. Switching monopolar radiofrequency ablation technique using multiple, internally cooled electrodes and a multichannel generator: ex vivo and in vivo pilot study. Investigative radiology. 2007 Mar;42(3):163-71.

[83] Laeseke PF, Sampson LA, Haemmerich D, Brace CL, Fine JP, Frey TM, et al. *Multiple-electrode radiofrequency ablation creates confluent areas of necrosis: in vivo porcine liver results.* Radiology. 2006 Oct;241(1):116-24.

[84] Bugge E, Nicholson IA, Thomas SP. *Comparison of bipolar and unipolar radiofrequency ablation in an in vivo experimental model.* Eur J Cardiothorac Surg. 2005 Jul;28(1):76-80; discussion -2.

[85] Frericks BB, Ritz JP, Roggan A, Wolf KJ, Albrecht T. *Multipolar radiofrequency ablation of hepatic tumors: initial experience.* Radiology. 2005 Dec;237(3):1056-62.

[86] Tacke J, Mahnken A, Roggan A, Gunther RW. *Multipolar radiofrequency ablation: first clinical results.* Rofo. 2004 Mar;176(3):324-9.

[87] Clasen S, Schmidt D, Boss A, Dietz K, Krober SM, Claussen CD, et al. *Multipolar radiofrequency ablation with internally cooled electrodes: experimental study in ex vivo bovine liver with mathematic modeling.* Radiology. 2006 Mar;238(3):881-90.

[88] Seror O, N'Kontchou G, Ibraheem M, Ajavon Y, Barrucand C, Ganne N, et al. *Large (>or=5.0-cm) HCCs: multipolar RF ablation with three internally cooled bipolar electrodes--initial experience in 26 patients.* Radiology. 2008 Jul;248(1):288-96.

[89] Lee JM, Han JK, Kim SH, Han CJ, An SK, Lee JY, et al. *Wet radiofrequency ablation using multiple electrodes: comparative study of bipolar versus monopolar modes in the bovine liver.* European journal of radiology. 2005 Jun;54(3):408-17.

[90] Lee JM, Han JK, Lee JY, Kim SH, Choi JY, Lee MW, et al. *Hepatic radiofrequency ablation using multiple probes: ex vivo and in vivo comparative studies of monopolar versus multipolar modes.* Korean J Radiol. 2006 Apr-Jun;7(2):106-17.

[91] Lee JM, Han JK, Kim HC, Kim SH, Kim KW, Joo SM, et al. *Multipleelectrode radiofrequency ablation of in vivo porcine liver: comparative studies of consecutive monopolar, switching monopolar versus multipolar modes.* Investigative radiology. 2007 Oct;42(10):676-83.

[92] Haemmerich D, Staelin ST, Tungjitkusolmun S, Lee FT, Jr., Mahvi DM, Webster JG. *Hepatic bipolar radio-frequency ablation between separated multiprong electrodes.* IEEE Trans Biomed Eng. 2001 Oct;48(10):1145-52.

[93] Livraghi T. *Treatment of hepatocellular carcinoma by interventional methods.* European radiology. 2001;11(11):2207-19.

[94] Crocetti L, de Baere T, Lencioni R. *Quality improvement guidelines for radiofrequency ablation of liver tumours.* Cardiovascular and interventional radiology. 2010 Feb;33(1):11-7.

[95] Chen MH, Yang W, Yan K, Zou MW, Solbiati L, Liu JB, et al. *Large liver tumors: protocol for radiofrequency ablation and its clinical application in 110 patients--mathematic model, overlapping mode, and electrode placement process.* Radiology. 2004 Jul;232(1):260-71.

[96] Rhim H, Dodd GD, 3rd, Chintapalli KN, Wood BJ, Dupuy DE, Hvizda JL, et al. *Radiofrequency thermal ablation of abdominal tumors: lessons learned from complications.* Radiographics. 2004 Jan-Feb;24(1):41-52.

[97] Livraghi T, Lazzaroni S, Meloni F, Solbiati L. *Risk of tumour seeding after percutaneous radiofrequency ablation for hepatocellular carcinoma.* The British journal of surgery. 2005 Jul;92(7):856-8.

[98] Rossi S, Di Stasi M, Buscarini E, Quaretti P, Garbagnati F, Squassante L, et al. *Percutaneous RF interstitial thermal ablation in the treatment of hepatic cancer.* Ajr. 1996 Sep;167(3):759-68.

[99] Nakai M, Sato M, Sahara S, Takasaka I, Kawai N, Minamiguchi H, et al. *Radiofrequency ablation assisted by real-time virtual sonography and CT*

for hepatocellular carcinoma undetectable by conventional sonography. Cardiovascular and interventional radiology. 2009 Jan;32(1):62-9.

[100] Livraghi T. *Radiofrequency ablation, PEIT, and TACE for hepatocellular carcinoma.* Journal of hepato-biliary-pancreatic surgery. 2003;10(1):67-76.

[101] Dodd GD, 3rd, Frank MS, Aribandi M, Chopra S, Chintapalli KN. *Radiofrequency thermal ablation: computer analysis of the size of the thermal injury created by overlapping ablations.* Ajr. 2001 Oct;177(4):777-82.

[102] Dodd GD, 3rd, Soulen MC, Kane RA, Livraghi T, Lees WR, Yamashita Y, et al. *Minimally invasive treatment of malignant hepatic tumors: at the threshold of a major breakthrough.* Radiographics. 2000 Jan-Feb;20(1):9-27.

[103] Widmann G, Bodner G, Bale R. *Tumour ablation: technical aspects.* Cancer Imaging. 2009;9 Spec No A:S63-7.

[104] Dominique E, El Otmany A, Goharin A, Attalah D, de Baere T. *Intraductal cooling of the main bile ducts during intraoperative radiofrequency ablation.* J Surg Oncol. 2001 Apr;76(4):297-300.

[105] Wood TF, Rose DM, Chung M, Allegra DP, Foshag LJ, Bilchik AJ. *Radiofrequency ablation of 231 unresectable hepatic tumors: indications, limitations, and complications.* Annals of surgical oncology. 2000 Sep;7(8):593-600.

[106] Chopra S, Dodd GD, 3rd, Chanin MP, Chintapalli KN. *Radiofrequency ablation of hepatic tumors adjacent to the gallbladder: feasibility and safety.* Ajr. 2003 Mar;180(3):697-701.

[107] Chen EA, Neeman Z, Lee FT, Kam A, Wood B. *Thermal protection with 5% dextrose solution blanket during radiofrequency ablation.* Cardiovascular and interventional radiology. 2006 Nov-Dec;29(6):1093-6.

[108] Kondo Y, Yoshida H, Shiina S, Tateishi R, Teratani T, Omata M. *Artificial ascites technique for percutaneous radiofrequency ablation of liver cancer adjacent to the gastrointestinal tract.* The British journal of surgery. 2006 Oct;93(10):1277-82.

[109] Laeseke PF, Sampson LA, Brace CL, Winter TC, 3rd, Fine JP, Lee FT, Jr. *Unintended thermal injuries from radiofrequency ablation: protection with 5% dextrose in water.* Ajr. 2006 May;186(5 Suppl):S249-54.

[110] Yamakado K, Nakatsuka A, Akeboshi M, Takeda K. *Percutaneous radiofrequency ablation of liver neoplasms adjacent to the gastrointestinal tract after balloon catheter interposition.* J Vasc Interv Radiol. 2003 Sep;14(9 Pt 1):1183-6.

CT-Guided Radiofrequency Ablation of Liver Tumors 65

[111] Kleinert R, Wahba R, Bangard C, Prenzel K, Holscher AH, Stippel D. *Radiomorphology of the Habib sealer-induced resection plane during long-time followup: a longitudinal single center experience after 64 radiofrequency-assisted liver resections.* HPB Surg. 2010;2010:403097.

[112] Akyildiz HY, Morris-Stiff G, Aucejo F, Fung J, Berber E. *Techniques of radiofrequency-assisted precoagulation in laparoscopic liver resection.* Surgical endoscopy. 2011 Apr;25(4):1143-7.

[113] Curro G, Bartolotta M, Barbera A, Jiao L, Habib N, Navarra G. *Ultrasound-guided radiofrequency-assisted segmental liver resection: a new technique.* Annals of surgery. 2009 Aug;250(2):229-33.

[114] Jiao LR, Ayav A, Navarra G, Sommerville C, Pai M, Damrah O, et al. *Laparoscopic liver resection assisted by the laparoscopic Habib Sealer.* Surgery. 2008 Nov;144(5):770-4.

[115] Pai M, Jiao LR, Khorsandi S, Canelo R, Spalding DR, Habib NA. *Liver resection with bipolar radiofrequency device: Habib 4X.* HPB (Oxford). 2008;10(4):256-60.

[116] Pai M, Navarra G, Ayav A, Sommerville C, Khorsandi SK, Damrah O, et al. *Laparoscopic Habib 4X: a bipolar radiofrequency device for bloodless laparoscopic liver resection.* HPB (Oxford). 2008;10(4):261-4.

[117] Weber JC, Navarra G, Jiao LR, Nicholls JP, Jensen SL, Habib NA. *New technique for liver resection using heat coagulative necrosis.* Annals of surgery. 2002 Nov;236(5):560-3.

[118] Ayav A, Jiao LR, Habib NA. *Bloodless liver resection using radiofrequency energy.* Digestive surgery. 2007;24(4):314-7.

[119] Ayav A, Navarra G, Basaglia E, Tierris J, Healey A, Spalding D, et al. *Results of major hepatectomy without vascular clamping using radiofrequency-assisted technique compared with total vascular exclusion.* Hepato-gastroenterology. 2007 Apr-May;54(75):806-9.

[120] Bachellier P, Ayav A, Pai M, Weber JC, Rosso E, Jaeck D, et al. *Laparoscopic liver resection assisted with radiofrequency.* Am J Surg. 2007 Apr;193(4):427-30.

[121] Livraghi T, Meloni F. *Removal of liver tumours using radiofrequency waves.* Annales chirurgiae et gynaecologiae. 2001;90(4):239-45.

[122] Livraghi T. *Guidelines for treatment of liver cancer.* Eur J Ultrasound. 2001 Jun;13(2):167-76.

[123] Bale R, Widmann G, Stoffner DI. *Stereotaxy: breaking the limits of current radiofrequency ablation techniques.* European journal of radiology. 2010 Jul;75(1):32-6.

[124] Mulier S, Ni Y, Jamart J, Ruers T, Marchal G, Michel L. *Local recurrence after hepatic radiofrequency coagulation: multivariate meta-analysis and review of contributing factors.* Annals of surgery. 2005 Aug;242(2):158-71.

[125] Livraghi T, Lazzaroni S, Meloni F. *Radiofrequency thermal ablation of hepatocellular carcinoma.* Eur J Ultrasound. 2001 Jun;13(2):159-66.

[126] Rhim H. *Complications of radiofrequency ablation in hepatocellular carcinoma.* Abdominal imaging. 2005 Jul-Aug;30(4):409-18.

[127] Rhim H, Lim HK. *Radiofrequency ablation for hepatocellular carcinoma abutting the diaphragm: the value of artificial ascites.* Abdominal imaging. 2009 May-Jun;34(3):371-80.

[128] Rhim H, Lee MH, Kim YS, Choi D, Lee WJ, Lim HK. *Planning sonography to assess the feasibility of percutaneous radiofrequency ablation of hepatocellular carcinomas.* Ajr. 2008 May;190(5):1324-30.

[129] Rhim H, Lim HK, Kim YS, Choi D. *Percutaneous radiofrequency ablation with artificial ascites for hepatocellular carcinoma in the hepatic dome: initial experience.* Ajr. 2008 Jan;190(1):91-8.

[130] Rode A, Bancel B, Douek P, Chevallier M, Vilgrain V, Picaud G, et al. *Small nodule detection in cirrhotic livers: evaluation with US, spiral CT, and MRI and correlation with pathologic examination of explanted liver.* J Comput Assist Tomogr. 2001 May-Jun;25(3):327-36.

[131] Minami Y, Chung H, Kudo M, Kitai S, Takahashi S, Inoue T, et al. *Radiofrequency ablation of hepatocellular carcinoma: value of virtual CT sonography with magnetic navigation.* Ajr. 2008 Jun;190(6):W335-41.

[132] Kruskal JB, Oliver B, Huertas JC, Goldberg SN. *Dynamic intrahepatic flow and cellular alterations during radiofrequency ablation of liver tissue in mice.* J Vasc Interv Radiol. 2001 Oct;12(10):1193-201.

[133] Cha CH, Lee FT, Jr., Gurney JM, Markhardt BK, Warner TF, Kelcz F, et al. *CT versus sonography for monitoring radiofrequency ablation in a porcine liver.* Ajr. 2000 Sep;175(3):705-11.

[134] Solbiati L, Ierace T, Goldberg SN, Sironi S, Livraghi T, Fiocca R, et al. *Percutaneous US-guided radio-frequency tissue ablation of liver metastases: treatment and follow-up in 16 patients.* Radiology. 1997 Jan;202(1):195-203.

[135] Meloni MF, Goldberg SN, Livraghi T, Calliada F, Ricci P, Rossi M, et al. *Hepatocellular carcinoma treated with radiofrequency ablation: comparison of pulse inversion contrast-enhanced harmonic sonography, contrast-enhanced power Doppler sonography, and helical CT.* Ajr. 2001 Aug;177(2):375-80.

CT-Guided Radiofrequency Ablation of Liver Tumors

[136] Minami Y, Kudo M, Kawasaki T, Chung H, Ogawa C, Shiozaki H. *Treatment of hepatocellular carcinoma with percutaneous radiofrequency ablation: usefulness of contrast harmonic sonography for lesions poorly defined with B-mode sonography.* Ajr. 2004 Jul;183(1):153-6.

[137] Raman SS, Lu DS, Vodopich DJ, Sayre J, Lassman C. *Creation of radiofrequency lesions in a porcine model: correlation with sonography, CT, and histopathology.* Ajr. 2000 Nov;175(5):1253-8.

[138] Leyendecker JR, Dodd GD, 3rd, Halff GA, McCoy VA, Napier DH, Hubbard LG, et al. *Sonographically observed echogenic response during intraoperative radiofrequency ablation of cirrhotic livers: pathologic correlation.* Ajr. 2002 May;178(5):1147-51.

[139] Claudon M, Cosgrove D, Albrecht T, Bolondi L, Bosio M, Calliada F, et al. *Guidelines and good clinical practice recommendations for contrast enhanced ultrasound (CEUS) - update 2008.* Ultraschall Med. 2008 Feb;29(1):28-44.

[140] Spinazzi A. *Emerging clinical applications for contrast-enhanced ultrasonography.* European radiology. 2001;11 Suppl 3:E7-12.

[141] Nicolau C, Bru C. *Focal liver lesions: evaluation with contrast-enhanced ultrasonography.* Abdominal imaging. 2004 May-Jun;29(3):348-59.

[142] Solbiati L, Tonolini M, Cova L, Goldberg SN. *The role of contrast-enhanced ultrasound in the detection of focal liver leasions.* European radiology. 2001;11 Suppl 3:E15-26.

[143] Leen E. *The role of contrast-enhanced ultrasound in the characterisation of focal liver lesions.* European radiology. 2001;11 Suppl 3:E27-34.

[144] Solbiati L, Ierace T, Tonolini M, Cova L. *Guidance and control of percutaneous treatments with contrast-enhanced ultrasound.* European radiology. 2003 Nov;13 Suppl 3:N87-90.

[145] Kim CK, Choi D, Lim HK, Kim SH, Lee WJ, Kim MJ, et al. *Therapeutic response assessment of percutaneous radiofrequency ablation for hepatocellular carcinoma: utility of contrast-enhanced agent detection imaging.* European journal of radiology. 2005 Oct;56(1):66-73.

[146] Albrecht T, Blomley M, Bolondi L, Claudon M, Correas JM, Cosgrove D, et al. *Guidelines for the use of contrast agents in ultrasound. January 2004.* Ultraschall Med. 2004 Aug;25(4):249-56.

[147] Minami Y, Kudo M, Chung H, Kawasaki T, Yagyu Y, Shimono T, et al. *Contrast harmonic sonography-guided radiofrequency ablation therapy versus B-mode sonography in hepatocellular carcinoma: prospective randomized controlled trial.* Ajr. 2007 Feb;188(2):489-94.

[148] Solbiati L, Goldberg SN, Ierace T, Dellanoce M, Livraghi T, Gazelle GS. *Radio-frequency ablation of hepatic metastases: postprocedural assessment with a US microbubble contrast agent--early experience.* Radiology. 1999 Jun;211(3):643-9.

[149] Lu MD, Yu XL, Li AH, Jiang TA, Chen MH, Zhao BZ, et al. *Comparison of contrast enhanced ultrasound and contrast enhanced CT or MRI in monitoring percutaneous thermal ablation procedure in patients with hepatocellular carcinoma: a multi-center study in China.* Ultrasound Med Biol. 2007 Nov;33(11):1736-49.

[150] Solbiati L, Ierace T, Tonolini M, Cova L. *Guidance and monitoring of radiofrequency liver tumor ablation with contrast-enhanced ultrasound.* European journal of radiology. 2004 Jun;51 Suppl:S19-23.

[151] Choi D, Lim HK, Lee WJ, Kim SH, Kim YH, Lim JH. *Early assessment of the therapeutic response to radio frequency ablation for hepatocellular carcinoma: utility of gray scale harmonic ultrasonography with a microbubble contrast agent.* J Ultrasound Med. 2003 Nov;22(11):1163-72.

[152] Kuehl H, Antoch G, Stergar H, Veit-Haibach P, Rosenbaum-Krumme S, Vogt F, et al. *Comparison of FDG-PET, PET/CT and MRI for follow-up of colorectal liver metastases treated with radiofrequency ablation: initial results.* European journal of radiology. 2008 Aug;67(2):362-71.

[153] Ba-Ssalamah A, Heinz-Peer G, Schima W, Schibany N, Schick S, Prokesch RW, et al. *Detection of focal hepatic lesions: comparison of unenhanced and SHU 555 A-enhanced MR imaging versus biphasic helical CTAP.* J Magn Reson Imaging. 2000 Jun;11(6):665-72.

[154] Ba-Ssalamah A, Schima W, Schmook MT, Linnau KF, Schibany N, Helbich T, et al. *Atypical focal nodular hyperplasia of the liver: imaging features of nonspecific and liver-specific MR contrast agents.* Ajr. 2002 Dec;179(6):1447-56.

[155] Schima W, Kulinna C, Langenberger H, Ba-Ssalamah A. *Liver metastases of colorectal cancer: US, CT or MR?* Cancer Imaging. 2005;5 Spec No A:S149-56.

[156] Trattnig S, Ba-Ssalamah A, Noebauer-Huhmann IM, Barth M, Wolfsberger S, Pinker K, et al. *MR contrast agent at high-field MRI (3 Tesla).* Top Magn Reson Imaging. 2003 Oct;14(5):365-75.

[157] Rosenkranz AR, Grobner T, Mayer GJ. *Conventional or Gadolinium containing contrast media: the choice between acute renal failure or Nephrogenic Systemic Fibrosis?* Wien Klin Wochenschr. 2007;119(9-10):271-5.

CT-Guided Radiofrequency Ablation of Liver Tumors 69

[158] Grobner T, Prischl FC. *Gadolinium and nephrogenic systemic fibrosis.* Kidney Int. 2007 Aug;72(3):260-4.

[159] Maeda T, Hong J, Konishi K, Nakatsuji T, Yasunaga T, Yamashita Y, et al. *Tumor ablation therapy of liver cancers with an open magnetic resonance imaging-based navigation system.* Surgical endoscopy. 2009 May;23(5):1048-53.

[160] Kettenbach J, Kacher DF, Koskinen SK, Silverman SG, Nabavi A, Gering D, et al. *Interventional and intraoperative magnetic resonance imaging.* Annual review of biomedical engineering. 2000;2:661-90.

[161] Blum M, Mueller C, Peck-Radosavljevic M, Wrba F, Berlakovich G, Muhlbacher F, et al. *MR-guided percutaneous ethanol ablation of hepatocellular carcinomas before liver transplantation.* Minim Invasive Ther Allied Technol. 2007;16(4):230-40.

[162] Clasen S, Boss A, Schmidt D, Schraml C, Fritz J, Schick F, et al. *MR-guided radiofrequency ablation in a 0.2-T open MR system: technical success and technique effectiveness in 100 liver tumors.* J Magn Reson Imaging. 2007 Oct;26(4):1043-52.

[163] McDannold NJ, Jolesz FA. *Magnetic resonance image-guided thermal ablations.* Top Magn Reson Imaging. 2000 Jun;11(3):191-202.

[164] Jantschke R, Haas T, Madoerin P, Dziergwa S. *Preparation, assistance and imaging protocols for robotically assisted MR and CT- based procedures.* Minim Invasive Ther Allied Technol. 2007;16(4):217-21.

[165] Kettenbach J, Kacher DF, Kanan AR, Rostenberg B, Fairhurst J, Stadler A, et al. *Intraoperative and interventional MRI: recommendations for a safe environment.* Minim Invasive Ther Allied Technol. 2006;15(2):53-64.

[166] de Senneville BD, Mougenot C, Quesson B, Dragonu I, Grenier N, Moonen CT. *MR thermometry for monitoring tumor ablation.* European radiology. 2007 Sep;17(9):2401-10.

[167] Seror O, Lepetit-Coiffe M, Le Bail B, de Senneville BD, Trillaud H, Moonen C, et al. *Real time monitoring of radiofrequency ablation based on MR thermometry and thermal dose in the pig liver in vivo.* European radiology. 2008 Feb;18(2):408-16.

[168] Clasen S, Pereira PL. *Magnetic resonance guidance for radiofrequency ablation of liver tumors.* J Magn Reson Imaging. 2008 Feb;27(2):421-33.

[169] Sironi S, Livraghi T, Meloni F, De Cobelli F, Ferrero C, Del Maschio A. *Small hepatocellular carcinoma treated with percutaneous RF ablation: MR imaging follow-up.* Ajr. 1999 Nov;173(5):1225-9.

[170] Willatt JM, Hussain HK, Adusumilli S, Marrero JA. MR *Imaging of hepatocellular carcinoma in the cirrhotic liver: challenges and controversies.* Radiology. 2008 May;247(2):311-30.

[171] Bluemke DA, Sahani D, Amendola M, Balzer T, Breuer J, Brown JJ, et al. *Efficacy and safety of MR imaging with liver-specific contrast agent: U.S. multicenter phase III study.* Radiology. 2005 Oct;237(1):89-98.

[172] Tanimoto A, Kuribayashi S. *Application of superparamagnetic iron oxide to imaging of hepatocellular carcinoma.* European journal of radiology. 2006 May;58(2):200-16.

[173] Tanimoto A, Mukai M, Kuribayashi S. *Evaluation of superparamagnetic iron oxide for MR imaging of liver injury: proton relaxation mechanisms and optimal MR imaging parameters.* Magn Reson Med Sci. 2006 Jul;5(2):89-98.

[174] Maluf DG, Stravitz RT, Williams B, Cotterell AH, Mas VR, Heuman D, et al. *Multimodality therapy and liver transplantation in patients with cirrhosis and hepatocellular carcinoma: 6 years, single-center experience.* Transplant Proc. 2007 Jan-Feb;39(1):153-9.

[175] Bale R, Widmann G. *Navigated CT-guided interventions.* Minim Invasive Ther Allied Technol. 2007;16(4):196-204.

[176] Jacob AL, Regazzoni P, Bilecen D, Rasmus M, Huegli RW, Messmer P. *Medical technology integration: CT, angiography, imaging-capable OR-table, navigation and robotics in a multifunctional sterile suite.* Minim Invasive Ther Allied Technol. 2007;16(4):205-11.

[177] Giesel FL, Mehndiratta A, Locklin J, McAuliffe MJ, White S, Choyke PL, et al. *Image fusion using CT, MRI and PET for treatment planning, navigation and follow up in percutaneous RFA.* Exp Oncol. 2009 Jun;31(2):106-14.

[178] Penney GP, Blackall JM, Hamady MS, Sabharwal T, Adam A, Hawkes DJ. *Registration of freehand 3D ultrasound and magnetic resonance liver images.* Medical image analysis. 2004 Mar;8(1):81-91.

[179] Hong J, Nakashima H, Konishi K, Ieiri S, Tanoue K, Nakamuta M, et al. *Interventional navigation for abdominal therapy based on simultaneous use of MRI and ultrasound.* Medical & biological engineering & computing. 2006 Dec;44(12):1127-34.

[180] Zhang H, Banovac F, Lin R, Glossop N, Wood BJ, Lindisch D, et al. *Electromagnetic tracking for abdominal interventions in computer aided surgery.* Comput Aided Surg. 2006 May;11(3):127-36.

[181] Lagana D, Carrafiello G, Mangini M, Lumia D, Mocciardini L, Chini C, et al. *Hepatic radiofrequency under CT-fluoroscopy guidance.* La Radiologia medica. 2008 Feb;113(1):87-100.

[182] Keil S, Bruners P, Ohnsorge L, Plumhans C, Behrendt FF, Stanzel S, et al. *Semiautomated versus manual evaluation of liver metastases treated by radiofrequency ablation.* J Vasc Interv Radiol. 2010 Feb;21(2):245-51.

[183] Keil S, Bruners P, Schiffl K, Sedlmair M, Muhlenbruch G, Gunther RW, et al. *Radiofrequency ablation of liver metastases-software-assisted evaluation of the ablation zone in MDCT: tumor-free follow-up versus local recurrent disease.* Cardiovascular and interventional radiology. 2010 Apr;33(2):297-306.

[184] Froelich JJ, Wagner HJ. *CT-fluoroscopy: Tool or gimmick?* Cardiovascular and interventional radiology. 2001 Sep-Oct;24(5):297-305.

[185] Silverman SG, Tuncali K, Adams DF, Nawfel RD, Zou KH, Judy PF. *CT fluoroscopy-guided abdominal interventions: techniques, results, and radiation exposure.* Radiology. 1999 Sep;212(3):673-81.

[186] Gusmao S, Oliveira M, Tazinaffo U, Honey CR. *Percutaneous trigeminal nerve radiofrequency rhizotomy guided by computerized tomography fluoroscopy.* Technical note. J Neurosurg. 2003 Oct;99(4):785-6.

[187] Teeuwisse WM, Geleijns J, Broerse JJ, Obermann WR, van Persijn van Meerten EL. *Patient and staff dose during CT guided biopsy, drainage and coagulation.* The British journal of radiology. 2001 Aug;74(884):720-6.

[188] Crocetti L, Lencioni R, Debeni S, See TC, Pina CD, Bartolozzi C. *Targeting liver lesions for radiofrequency ablation: an experimental feasibility study using a CT-US fusion imaging system.* Investigative radiology. 2008 Jan;43(1):33-9.

[189] Brabrand K, Aalokken TM, Krombach GA, Gunther RW, Tariq R, Magnusson A, et al. *Multicenter evaluation of a new laser guidance system for computed tomography intervention.* Acta Radiol. 2004 May;45(3):308-12.

[190] Varro Z, Locklin JK, Wood BJ. *Laser navigation for radiofrequency ablation.* Cardiovascular and interventional radiology. 2004 Sep-Oct;27(5):512-5.

[191] Pereles FS, Ozgur HT, Lund PJ, Unger EC. *Potentials of a new laser guidance system for percutaneous musculoskeletal procedures.* Skeletal radiology. 1998 Jan;27(1):18-21.

[192] Pereles FS, Baker M, Baldwin R, Krupinski E, Unger EC. *Accuracy of CT biopsy: laser guidance versus conventional freehand techniques.* Academic radiology. 1998 Nov;5(11):766-70.

[193] Meyer JM, Schmitz-Rode T, Krombach G, Wildberger JE, Pfeffer J, Gunther RW. *Navi-ball: a new guidance device for CT-directed punctures.* Investigative radiology. 2001 May;36(5):299-302.

[194] Magnusson A, Radecka E, Lonnemark M, Raland H. *Computed-tomography-guided punctures using a new guidance device.* Acta Radiol. 2005 Aug;46(5):505-9.

[195] West JB, Maurer CR, Jr. *Designing optically tracked instruments for image-guided surgery.* IEEE Trans Med Imaging. 2004 May;23(5):533-45.

[196] Kisaka Y, Hirooka M, Koizumi Y, Abe M, Matsuura B, Hiasa Y, et al. *Contrast-enhanced sonography with abdominal virtual sonography in monitoring radiofrequency ablation of hepatocellular carcinoma.* J Clin Ultrasound. 2010 Mar-Apr;38(3):138-44.

[197] Schweikard A, Shiomi H, Adler J. *Respiration tracking in radiosurgery.* Medical physics. 2004 Oct;31(10):2738-41.

[198] West JB, Fitzpatrick JM, Toms SA, Maurer CR, Jr., Maciunas RJ. *Fiducial point placement and the accuracy of point-based, rigid body registration.* Neurosurgery. 2001 Apr;48(4):810-6; discussion 6-7.

[199] Grunert P, Darabi K, Espinosa J, Filippi R. *Computer-aided navigation in neurosurgery.* Neurosurg Rev. 2003 May;26(2):73-99; discussion 100-1.

[200] Khan MF, Dogan S, Maataoui A, Wesarg S, Gurung J, Ackermann H, et al. *Navigation-based needle puncture of a cadaver using a hybrid tracking navigational system.* Investigative radiology. 2006 Oct;41(10):713-20.

[201] Lencioni R, Della Pina C, Bartolozzi C. *Percutaneous image-guided radiofrequency ablation in the therapeutic management of hepatocellular carcinoma.* Abdominal imaging. 2005 Jul-Aug;30(4):401-8.

[202] Ng KK, Lo CM, Liu CL, Poon RT, Chan SC, Fan ST. *Survival analysis of patients with transplantable recurrent hepatocellular carcinoma: implications for salvage liver transplant.* Arch Surg. 2008 Jan;143(1):68-74; discussion

[203] Okuwaki Y, Nakazawa T, Shibuya A, Ono K, Hidaka H, Watanabe M, et al. *Intrahepatic distant recurrence after radiofrequency ablation for a single small hepatocellular carcinoma: risk factors and patterns.* Journal of gastroenterology. 2008;43(1):71-8.

[204] Widmann G, Schullian P, Haidu M, Wiedermann FJ, Bale R. *Respiratory motion control for stereotactic and robotic liver interventions.* Int J Med Robot. 2010 Sep;6(3):343-9.

[205] Widmann G, Schullian P, Haidu M, Fasser M, Bale R. *Targeting accuracy of CT-guided stereotaxy for radiofrequency ablation of liver tumours.*

Minim Invasive Ther Allied Technol. 2011;2011 Apr 6. [Epub ahead of print].

[206] Bale RJ, Lottersberger C, Vogele M, Prassl A, Czermak B, Dessl A, et al. *A novel vacuum device for extremity immobilisation during digital angiography: preliminary clinical experiences.* European radiology. 2002 Dec;12(12):2890-4.

[207] Bale RJ, Vogele M, Rieger M, Buchberger W, Lukas P, Jaschke W. *A new vacuum device for extremity immobilization.* Ajr. 1999 Apr;172(4):1093-4.

[208] Nagel M, Schmidt G, Petzold R, Kalender WA. *A navigation system for minimally invasive CT-guided interventions.* Med Image Comput Comput Assist Interv Int Conf Med Image Comput Comput Assist Interv. 2005;8(Pt 2):33-40.

[209] Schweikard A, Glosser G, Bodduluri M, Murphy MJ, Adler JR. *Robotic motion compensation for respiratory movement during radiosurgery.* Comput Aided Surg. 2000;5(4):263-77.

[210] Banovac F, Tang J, Xu S, Lindisch D, Chung HY, Levy EB, et al. *Precision targeting of liver lesions using a novel electromagnetic navigation device in physiologic phantom and swine.* Medical physics. 2005 Aug;32(8):2698-705.

[211] Maier-Hein L, Muller SA, Pianka F, Worz S, Muller-Stich BP, Seitel A, et al. *Respiratory motion compensation for CT-guided interventions in the liver.* Comput Aided Surg. 2008 May;13(3):125-38.

[212] Maier-Hein L, Tekbas A, Seitel A, Pianka F, Muller SA, Satzl S, et al. *In vivo accuracy assessment of a needle-based navigation system for CT-guided radiofrequency ablation of the liver.* Medical physics. 2008 Dec;35(12):5385-96.

[213] Archip N, Tatli S, Morrison P, Jolesz F, Warfield SK, Silverman S. *Non-rigid registration of pre-procedural MR images with intra-procedural unenhanced CT images for improved targeting of tumors during liver radiofrequency ablations.* Med Image Comput Comput Assist Interv. 2007;10(Pt 2):969-77.

[214] Crum WR, Hartkens T, Hill DL. *Non-rigid image registration: theory and practice.* The British journal of radiology. 2004;77 Spec No 2:S140-53.

[215] Hutton BF, Braun M. *Software for image registration: algorithms, accuracy, efficacy.* Semin Nucl Med. 2003 Jul;33(3):180-92.

[216] Hill DL, Batchelor PG, Holden M, Hawkes DJ. *Medical image registration.* Phys Med Biol. 2001 Mar;46(3):R1-45.

[217] Widmann G. *Image-guided surgery and medical robotics in the cranial area.* Biomed Imaging Interv J. 2007;3(1):e11.

[218] Khadem R, Yeh CC, Sadeghi-Tehrani M, Bax MR, Johnson JA, Welch JN, et al. *Comparative tracking error analysis of five different optical tracking systems*. Comput Aided Surg. 2000;5(2):98-107.

[219] Watzinger F, Birkfellner W, Wanschitz F, Millesi W, Schopper C, Sinko K, et al. *Positioning of dental implants using computer-aided navigation and an optical tracking system: case report and presentation of a new method*. J Craniomaxillofac Surg. 1999 Apr;27(2):77-81.

[220] Widmann G, Stoffner R, Bale R. *Errors and error management in image-guided craniomaxillofacial surgery*. Oral surgery, oral medicine, oral pathology, oral radiology, and endodontics. 2009 May;107(5):701-15.

[221] Schiemann M, Killmann R, Kleen M, Abolmaali N, Finney J, Vogl TJ. *Vascular guide wire navigation with a magnetic guidance system: experimental results in a phantom*. Radiology. 2004 Aug;232(2):475-81.

[222] Banovac F, Glossop, N., Lindisch, D., Tanaka, D., Levy, E., Cleary, K., editor. *Liver tummor biopsy in a respiratory phantom with assistance of a novel electromagnetic navigation device*. MICCAI; 2002: Springer-Verlag Berlin Heidelberg 2002.

[223] Wood BJ, Zhang H, Durrani A, Glossop N, Ranjan S, Lindisch D, et al. *Navigation with electromagnetic tracking for interventional radiology procedures: a feasibility study*. J Vasc Interv Radiol. 2005 Apr;16(4):493-505.

[224] Wagner A, Schicho K, Birkfellner W, Figl M, Seemann R, Konig F, et al. *Quantitative analysis of factors affecting intraoperative precision and stability of optoelectronic and electromagnetic tracking systems*. Medical physics. 2002 May;29(5):905-12.

[225] Hummel J, Figl M, Birkfellner W, Bax MR, Shahidi R, Maurer CR, Jr., et al. *Evaluation of a new electromagnetic tracking system using a standardized assessment protocol*. Phys Med Biol. 2006 May 21;51(10):N205-10.

[226] Marmulla R, Hilbert M, Niederdellmann H. *[Intraoperative precision of mechanical, electromagnetic, infrared and laser-guided navigation systems in computer-assisted surgery]*. Mund Kiefer Gesichtschir. 1998 May;2 Suppl 1:S145-8.

[227] Gunkel AR, Freysinger W, Thumfart WF. *Experience with various 3-dimensional navigation systems in head and neck surgery*. Arch Otolaryngol Head Neck Surg. 2000 Mar;126(3):390-5.

[228] Birkfellner W, Watzinger F, Wanschitz F, Enislidis G, Kollmann C, Rafolt D, et al. *Systematic distortions in magnetic position digitizers*. Medical physics. 1998 Nov;25(11):2242-8.

[229] Mascott CR. *Comparison of magnetic tracking and optical tracking by simultaneous use of two independent frameless stereotactic systems.* Neurosurgery. 2005 Oct;57(4 Suppl):295-301; discussion 295-301.

[230] Koele W, Stammberger H, Lackner A, Reittner P. *Image guided surgery of paranasal sinuses and anterior skull base--five years experience with the InstaTrak-System.* Rhinology. 2002 Mar;40(1):1-9.

[231] Das M, Sauer F, Schoepf UJ, Khamene A, Vogt SK, Schaller S, et al. *Augmented reality visualization for CT-guided interventions: system description, feasibility, and initial evaluation in an abdominal phantom.* Radiology. 2006 Jul;240(1):230-5.

[232] Maier-Hein L, Tekbas A, Franz AM, Tetzlaff R, Muller SA, Pianka F, et al. *On combining internal and external fiducials for liver motion compensation.* Comput Aided Surg. 2008 Nov;13(6):369-76.

[233] Krucker J, Xu S, Glossop N, Viswanathan A, Borgert J, Schulz H, et al. *Electromagnetic tracking for thermal ablation and biopsy guidance: clinical evaluation of spatial accuracy.* J Vasc Interv Radiol. 2007 Sep;18(9):1141-50.

[234] Jacob AL, Messmer P, Kaim A, Suhm N, Regazzoni P, Baumann B. *A whole-body registration-free navigation system for image-guided surgery and interventional radiology.* Investigative radiology. 2000 May;35(5):279-88.

[235] Messmer P, Baumann B, Suhm N, Jacob AL. *[Navigation systems for image-guided therapy: A review].* Rofo. 2001 Sep;173(9):777-84.

[236] Messmer P, Gross T, Suhm N, Regazzoni P, Jacob AL, Huegli RW. *Modality-based navigation.* Injury. 2004 Jun;35 Suppl 1:S-A24-9.

[237] Levy EB, Tang J, Lindisch D, Glossop N, Banovac F, Cleary K. *Implementation of an electromagnetic tracking system for accurate intrahepatic puncture needle guidance: accuracy results in an in vitro model.* Academic radiology. 2007 Mar;14(3):344-54.

[238] Gralla J, Nimsky C, Buchfelder M, Fahlbusch R, Ganslandt O. *Frameless stereotactic brain biopsy procedures using the Stealth Station: indications, accuracy and results.* Zentralbl Neurochir. 2003;64(4):166-70.

[239] Barnett GH, Miller DW, Weisenberger J. *Frameless stereotaxy with scalp-applied fiducial markers for brain biopsy procedures: experience in 218 cases.* J Neurosurg. 1999 Oct;91(4):569-76.

[240] Bale RJ, Laimer I, Martin A, Schlager A, Mayr C, Rieger M, et al. *Frameless stereotactic cannulation of the foramen ovale for ablative treatment of trigeminal neuralgia.* Neurosurgery. 2006 Oct;59(4 Suppl 2):ONS394-401; discussion ONS2.

[241] Ortler M, Widmann G, Trinka E, Fiegele T, Eisner W, Twerdy K, et al. *Frameless stereotactic placement of foramen ovale electrodes in patients with drug-refractory temporal lobe epilepsy.* Neurosurgery. 2008 May;62(5 Suppl 2):ONS481-8; discussion ONS8-9.

[242] Dorward NL, Alberti O, Dijkstra A, Buurman J, Kitchen ND, Thomas DG. *Clinical introduction of an adjustable rigid instrument holder for frameless stereotactic interventions.* Comput Aided Surg. 1997;2(3-4):180-5.

[243] Dorward NL, Alberti O, Palmer JD, Kitchen ND, Thomas DG. *Accuracy of true frameless stereotaxy: in vivo measurement and laboratory phantom studies.* Technical note. J Neurosurg. 1999 Jan;90(1):160-8.

[244] Dorward NL, Paleologos TS, Alberti O, Thomas DG. *The advantages of frameless stereotactic biopsy over frame-based biopsy.* Br J Neurosurg. 2002 Apr;16(2):110-8.

[245] Stoffner R, Augscholl C, Widmann G, Bohler D, Bale R. *Accuracy and feasibility of frameless stereotactic and robot-assisted CT-based puncture in interventional radiology: a comparative phantom study.* Rofo. 2009 Sep;181(9):851-8.

[246] Widmann G, Eisner W, Kovacs P, Fiegele T, Ortler M, Lang TB, et al. *Accuracy and clinical use of a novel aiming device for frameless stereotactic brain biopsy.* Minim Invasive Neurosurg. 2008 Dec;51(6):361-9.

[247] Ortler M, Unterhofer C, Bauer R, Dobesberger J, Trinka E, Bale R. *Flexibility of head positioning and head fixation provided by a novel system for non-invasive maxillary fixation and frameless stereotaxy: technical note.* Minim Invasive Neurosurg. 2009 Jun;52(3):144-8.

[248] Ortler M, Trinka E, Dobesberger J, Bauer R, Unterhofer C, Twerdy K, et al. *Integration of multimodality imaging and surgical navigation in the management of patients with refractory epilepsy. A pilot study using a new minimally invasive reference and head-fixation system.* Acta neurochirurgica. 2010 Feb;152(2):365-78.

[249] Mehta AD, Labar D, Dean A, Harden C, Hosain S, Pak J, et al. *Frameless stereotactic placement of depth electrodes in epilepsy surgery.* J Neurosurg. 2005 Jun;102(6):1040-5.

[250] Cleary K, Melzer A, Watson V, Kronreif G, Stoianovici D. *Interventional robotic systems: applications and technology state-of-the-art.* Minim Invasive Ther Allied Technol. 2006;15(2):101-13.

[251] Cleary K, Nguyen C. *State of the art in surgical robotics: clinical applications and technology challenges.* Comput Aided Surg. 2001;6(6):312-28.

CT-Guided Radiofrequency Ablation of Liver Tumors 77

[252] Kettenbach J, Kronreif G, Figl M, Furst M, Birkfellner W, Hanel R, et al. *Robot-assisted biopsy using computed tomography-guidance: initial results from in vitro tests.* Investigative radiology. 2005 Apr;40(4):219-28.

[253] Rasmus M, Huegli RW, Bilecen D, Jacob AL. *Robotically assisted CT-based procedures.* Minim Invasive Ther Allied Technol. 2007;16(4):212-6.

[254] Fujioka C, Horiguchi J, Ishifuro M, Kakizawa H, Kiguchi M, Matsuura N, et al. *A feasibility study: evaluation of radiofrequency ablation therapy to hepatocellular carcinoma using image registration of preoperative and postoperative CT.* Academic radiology. 2006 Aug;13(8):986-94.

[255] Rhim H. *Sonography versus CT for monitoring radiofrequency ablation.* Ajr. 2001 Apr;176(4):1077-8.

[256] Catalano O, Esposito M, Nunziata A, Siani A. *Multiphase helical CT findings after percutaneous ablation procedures for hepatocellular carcinoma.* Abdominal imaging. 2000 Nov-Dec;25(6):607-14.

[257] Park MH, Rhim H, Kim YS, Choi D, Lim HK, Lee WJ. *Spectrum of CT findings after radiofrequency ablation of hepatic tumors.* Radiographics. 2008 Mar-Apr;28(2):379-90; discussion 90-2.

[258] Schraml C, Clasen S, Schwenzer NF, Koenigsrainer I, Herberts T, Claussen CD, et al. *Diagnostic performance of contrast-enhanced computed tomography in the immediate assessment of radiofrequency ablation success in colorectal liver metastases.* Abdominal imaging. 2008 Nov-Dec;33(6):643-51.

[259] Frich L, Hagen G, Brabrand K, Edwin B, Mathisen O, Aalokken TM, et al. *Local tumor progression after radiofrequency ablation of colorectal liver metastases: evaluation of ablative margin and three-dimensional volumetric analysis.* J Vasc Interv Radiol. 2007 Sep;18(9):1134-40.

[260] Lim HK, Choi D, Lee WJ, Kim SH, Lee SJ, Jang HJ, et al. *Hepatocellular carcinoma treated with percutaneous radio-frequency ablation: evaluation with follow-up multiphase helical CT.* Radiology. 2001 Nov;221(2):447-54.

[261] Vogt FM, Antoch G, Veit P, Freudenberg LS, Blechschmid N, Diersch O, et al. *Morphologic and functional changes in nontumorous liver tissue after radiofrequency ablation in an in vivo model: comparison of 18F-FDG PET/CT, MRI, ultrasound, and CT.* J Nucl Med. 2007 Nov;48(11):1836-44.

[262] Eisenhauer EA, Therasse P, Bogaerts J, Schwartz LH, Sargent D, Ford R, et al. *New response evaluation criteria in solid tumours: revised RECIST guideline (version 1.1).* Eur J Cancer. 2009 Jan;45(2):228-47.

[263] Lencioni R, Llovet JM. *Modified RECIST (mRECIST) assessment for hepatocellular carcinoma.* Semin Liver Dis. 2010 Feb;30(1):52-60.

[264] Nishino M, Jagannathan JP, Ramaiya NH, Van den Abbeele AD. *Revised RECIST guideline version 1.1: What oncologists want to know and what radiologists need to know.* Ajr. 2010 Aug;195(2):281-9.

[265] Massoptier L, Casciaro S. *A new fully automatic and robust algorithm for fast segmentation of liver tissue and tumors from CT scans.* European radiology. 2008 Aug;18(8):1658-65.

[266] Veit P, Antoch G, Stergar H, Bockisch A, Forsting M, Kuehl H. *Detection of residual tumor after radiofrequency ablation of liver metastasis with dual-modality PET/CT: initial results.* European radiology. 2006 Jan;16(1):80-7.

[267] Halpern BS, Dahlbom M, Auerbach MA, Schiepers C, Fueger BJ, Weber WA, et al. *Optimizing imaging protocols for overweight and obese patients: a lutetium orthosilicate PET/CT study.* J Nucl Med. 2005 Apr;46(4):603-7.

[268] Lubezky N, Metser U, Geva R, Nakache R, Shmueli E, Klausner JM, et al. *The role and limitations of 18-fluoro-2-deoxy-D-glucose positron emission tomography (FDG-PET) scan and computerized tomography (CT) in restaging patients with hepatic colorectal metastases following neoadjuvant chemotherapy: comparison with operative and pathological findings.* J Gastrointest Surg. 2007 Apr;11(4):472-8.

In: CT Scans
Editors: V. E. Perkel et al.

ISBN 978-1-62100-319-9
©2012 Nova Science Publishers, Inc.

Chapter 2

CARDIAC COMPUTED TOMOGRAPHY IMAGING: AN UPDATE ON PROCEDURES, APPLICATIONS AND HEALTH RISKS

Ali Ahmad, John F. Heitner and Igor Mamkin
New York Methodist Hospital, NY, U. S.

INTRODUCTION

Computed tomography (CT) is an imaging technique that has revolutionized medical imaging: it is widely available, fast, and provides a detailed view of the internal organs and structures. There are two types of CT scanners available, the conventional step and shoot (axial) and the helical CT. Axial CT is used for high resolution imaging of the lungs, coronary calcium scoring, and prospective ECG-gated coronary angiography. The two main components of CT scanners are the x-ray tube and a diametrically opposed array of detectors. The X-ray tube rotates around the patient and generates an X-ray beam and the detectors concurrently record the radiation that traverses the body while rejecting the scattered radiation emanating from outside the X-ray tube focal spot (the area of the target of the X-ray tube).

The introduction of multislice CT was a major technical advance in helical CT scanning. During multislice helical CT, a cone shaped X-ray beam (wider collimation than the conventional fan shaped X-ray beam) strikes many of the detector rows (4-320) that are arranged in parallel along the longitudinal axis (i.e., along the direction of the table motion. (Figure 1) The combination of a cone shaped X-ray beam and multiple rows of detectors allow a larger proportion of the X-ray beam to be used for imaging; multiple channels extract the data that are obtained simultaneously from different anatomic sections.

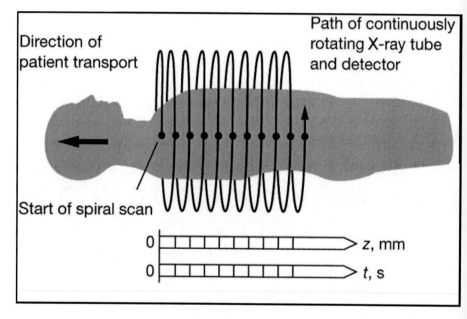

Figure 1. The scanning principle of single-spiral CT. In a multiple-spiral CT, such as a 4-detector-row CT, the helix in the schematic would be a quadruple helix that covers four times the distance in one turn. (Reproduced with permission).

CARDIAC CT TECHNOLOGY AND IMAGING OF THE HEART

Imaging of the heart and coronary arteries with CT is complicated by the rapid non-linear motion of the cardiac structures and was not feasible prior to the introduction of ECG-gating and multislice technology. Multislice technology carries the following advantages over conventional helical CT:

1) It is faster, with several hundred slices generated in 60 seconds or less, which allows for a complete cardiac scan in one cardiac cycle (if the heart rate is appropriate).
2) Its 360-degree reconstruction algorithm reduces signal noise by a factor of 1.4 compared to the 180-degree reconstruction algorithm that is used in single slice helical CT. signal noise in its simplest

definition is measured as the standard deviation of voxel values in a homogenous phantom (typically water) and is affected with multiple factors including the exposure time, collimation/reconstructed slice thickness, reconstruction algorithm, helical pitch and table speed.

3) The temporal resolution is improved, with faster image acquisition and fewer motion artifacts.

4) The spatial resolution and Z-axis resolution are both improved, allowing nearly isotropic voxels.

5) Retrospective reconstruction can be performed without the need for additional data acquisition; virtually any thickness can be reconstructed, as long as the initial data set was acquired with a 0.5 mm to 0.65 mm detector width.

6) Improved contrast enhancement with enhanced conspicuity of vascular structures.

7) Enhanced image processing includes volume rendering, maximum intensity projections (MIP), shaded surface display, curved multi-planar reformation and virtual reality imaging.

Multislice CT constitutes the major CT imaging modality to visualize cardiac structures and coronary arteries. These multislice scanners use mechanically rotating gantries. Scanners from different manufacturers vary slightly in their technical specifications but all have two features in common: a temporal resolution high enough to allow imaging of the beating heart without motion artifact if the heart rate is slow and regular ($\leq$ 65 beats/min); and acquisition of more than one image slice per gantry rotation. Recent scanners now acquire at least 64 slices (also known as rows) simultaneously with a collimation of 0.6 mm with a gantry rotation time of 333 msec (corresponding to a temporal resolution of approximately 167 msec). The newest single-source MSCCT scanners, scanners with single X-ray tube, can acquire 256 or 312 slices with each gantry rotation. Dual source/dual energy scanners are also available which effectively improves temporal resolution by 50 percent (83 msec), thereby facilitating imaging without the need for beta-adrenergic receptor blockers.

Another form of CT imaging of the heart is the electron beam cardiac tomography (EBCT). This ultrafast CT uses an electron gun instead of an X-ray tube and detector array. An anode is bombarded by electrons producing an X-ray beam that sweeps the patient. Images are obtained in 50-100 milliseconds, essentially freezing motion. This modality is used mainly for coronary calcium scoring, details of this form of CT is beyond the scope of this chapter.

OPTIMIZING CARDIAC IMAGING

Image quality in cardiac CT is paramount to reach accurate diagnosis with the aim to scan the heart with little or no motion artifact together with optimal visualization of vascular structures. One important principle is to reduce the heart rate to less than 65 beats per minute using oral or intravenous beta-adrenergic receptor blockers. Nitroglycerin (typically 2 sub-lingual sprays) is typically given immediately before the scan to achieve coronary vasodilation. Calcium channel blockers may be considered as an alternative to beta-adrenergic receptor blockers in asthmatic patients or in patients with atrial fibrillation. Unlike beta-adrenergic receptor blocker, calcium channel blockers do not induce bronchospasm. However they are not as effective as beta blockers in slowing ventricular rate in patients with atrial fibrillation. If calcium channel blocker is to be used during cardiac CT imaging, diltiazem may be preferred because this drug demonstrates the least negative inotropic effect among the commonly used calcium channel blocker. If intravenous calcium channel blocker is used, the patient has to be closely monitored as this may induce hypotension particularly when given with nitrates. Occasionally intravenous lidocaine is used for ectopy suppression.

The timing and rate of injection of contrast medium is important. Synchronization of data acquisition and contrast enhancement can be achieved by calculating the veno-arterial transit time, using a small bolus of contrast agent and retrospective analysis of the enhancement pattern over time (so-called 'test bolus' technique), or by real-time monitoring of the arrival of the bolus, for example, in the ascending aorta (so-called 'bolus tracking' technique). Typically, the amount of contrast material required for coronary CT angiography is about 60–100 mL depending on scanner type, patient size, heart rate, and body mass index. The contrast agent should be of high iodine concentration. Usually, the flow rate is 5 mL/s, but especially in obese patients, increasing the flow rate may be advantageous.

After acquisition of the raw data, retrospective ECG-gated image data sets are generated. These data sets usually consist of 200–300 overlapping slices, 0.5–0.75 mm thick, in trans-axial orientation. For coronary artery imaging, it is important to carefully identify the time in the cardiac cycle,which shows the least cardiac motion. For lower heart rates, the best time is usually in the mid- to end-diastolic phase (70-75% of R-R interval), whereas for higher heart

Cardiac Computed Tomography Imaging

rates, reconstruction in end-systole may yield superior results. The average heart rate and heart rate variability have been shown to substantially influence image quality. The most important predictors for diagnostic image quality are a low (≤ 60 beats per minute.) and regular cardiac rhythm with minimal heart rate variability.

The following patient-related factors can interfere with the diagnostic quality of MSCCT:

1) Heart rate greater than 60 or 70 beats per minute
2) Irregular heart rhythm (atrial fibrillation or frequent atrial or ventricular extrasystole)
3) Inability to sustain a breath hold for at least 5 to 10 seconds
4) Severe coronary calcification or the presence of coronary artery stents, since image reconstruction artifacts related to radiodense material such as calcium or metal can obscure the coronary artery lumen.
5) Segments with a diameter <1.5 mm can usually not be assessed for stenosis. Such small vessel caliber is typical of distal coronary artery segments and some side branches.
6) It can't be used in patient with allergy to contrast media or in patients at risk of contrast induced nephropathy.

CLINICAL UTILITY OF MSCCT

A. Coronary Artery Imaging

A number of studies have examined the diagnostic accuracy of MSCCT for detecting coronary artery stenoses. Most studies published to date are single center studies that describe the findings of experienced observers in relatively small number of patients who were referred for CT coronary angiography and had a relatively high prevalence of disease. The diagnostic accuracy that can be expected among patient populations with a lower prevalence of disease or from less experienced observers is not known. Another important observation in these studies is that they used invasive coronary angiography as the gold standard with >50% stenosis as a definition of significant stenosis. However, stenoses of less than 70 percent are typically not flow-limiting, are rarely the cause of ischemia or angina, and usually do not require revascularization. Thus, the sensitivities reported in the literature may not accurately reflect the ability of MSCCT to identify those patients with chest pain who will need catheter-based or surgical revascularization.

The results of recent studies that analyzed the accuracy of 64-slice CT and dual-source CT for the detection of coronary artery stenoses in patients with suspected coronary artery disease (CAD) are summarized in Tables 1 and 2. Pooling the data of more than 800 patients yields a sensitivity of 89% (95% CI 87–90) with a specificity of 96% (95% CI 96–97) and a positive and negative predictive values of 78% (95% CI 76–80) and 98% (95% CI 98–99), respectively. On average, 4.5% of segments (mainly distal segments or very small side branches) could not be evaluated. Importantly, the negative predictive value was consistently high in all studies, indicating that the technique may be most suitable as a non-invasive tool to rule out significant CAD and avoid further imaging or invasive angiography.

Three multicenter studies evaluated the diagnostic accuracy of 64-slice MSCCT for detection of significant (at least 50 percent diameter stenosis) coronary artery disease on quantitative invasive x-ray coronary angiography.

In the multicenter, single vendor, US based ACCURACY trial, 230 (94 percent) of 245 enrolled subjects completed the study protocol and all scans were evaluated visually. Patient-based sensitivity and specificity of MSCCT were 95 percent and 83 percent, respectively. Specificity fell to 53 percent for patients with calcium scores >400 Agatston units. In the multicenter, single vendor international CORE 64 study, 291 (72 percent) of 405 enrolled patients were eligible for analysis, calcium scores of ≤600 and able to complete the protocol. The patient-based sensitivity and specificity of MSCCT were 85 percent and 90 percent, respectively.

In a multicenter, multivendor study performed in the Netherlands, 360 (97 percent) of 371 enrolled patients completed the protocol. Patient-based sensitivity and specificity were 99 percent and 64 percent, respectively.

It is important to realize that patient selection may heavily influence results, with substantially impaired image quality in patients with higher heart rates or arrhythmias. Image quality may also be degraded in patients with extensive calcifications which potentially limit precise assessment of stenosis severity. Improvements can be expected with the introduction of dual-source CT systems, which provide higher temporal resolution by employing two rotating X-ray tubes rather than one. Preliminary studies using this technique showed that up to 98% of all coronary segments could be visualized without motion artifacts, even without lowering the heart rate by administration of beta-adrenergic receptor blockers. [35] Moreover, even in patients without a regular rhythm a high accuracy can be obtained.

Cardiac Computed Tomography Imaging

Table 1. Diagnostic performance of 64-slice computed tomography and dual-source computed tomography for the detection of significant coronary stenosis (luminal diameter >50%) on a per-segment basis (Reproduced with permission)

Author	Number of patients	Not evaluable (%)	Sensitivity (%)	Specificity (%)	PPV (%)	NPV (%)
Leschka et al.	67	0 (0/1005)	94 (165/176)	97 (805/829)	87 (165/189)	99 (805/816)
Leber et al.	55	0 (0/732)	76 (57/75)	97 (638/657)	75 (57/76)	97 (638/656)
Raff et al.	70	12 (130/1065)	86 (79/92)	95 (802/843)	76 (93/123)	99 (601/602)
Mollet et al.	51	0 (0/725)	99 (93/94)	95 (601/631)	76 (93/123)	99 (601/602)
Ropers et al.	81	4 (45/1128)	93 (39/42)	97 (1010/1041)	56 (39/70)	100 (1010/1013)
Schuijf et al.	60	1.4 (12/854)	85 (62/73)	98 (755/769)	82 (62/76)	99 (755/766)
Ong et al.	134	9.7 (143/1474)	82 (177/217)	96 (1067/1114)	79 (177/224)	96 (1067/1107)
Ehara et al.	69	8 (82/966)	90 (275/304)	94 (545/580)	89 (275/310)	95 (545/574)
Nikolaou et al.	72	9.5 (97/1020)	82 (97/118)	95 (762/805)	69 (97/140)	97 (762/789)
Weustink et al.	77	0 (0/1489)	95 (208/220)	95 (1200/1269)	75 (208/277)	99 (1200/1212)
Leber et al.	88	1.3 (16/1232)	94 (38/42)	99 (1165/1174)	81 (38/47)	99 (1165/1169)
Total	824	4.5 (525/11690) (95% CI 4.1–4.9)	89 (1290/1453) (95% CI 87–90)	96 (9350/9712) (95% CI 96–97)	78 (1290/1652) (95% CI 76–80)	98 (6350/9513) (95% CI 98–99)

All values are expressed as per cent with absolute numbers in parentheses. Sensitivity and specificity were calculated only for evaluable segments.
95% CI, 95% confidence interval; NPV, negative predictive value; PPV, positive predictive value.

Table 2. Diagnostic performance of 64-slice computed tomography and dual-source computed tomography for the detection of significant coronary stenosis (luminal diameter >50%) on a per-patient basis (Reproduced with permission)

Author	Number of patients	Not evaluable (%)	Sensitivity (%)	Specificity (%)	PPV (%)	NPV (%)
Leschka et al.	67	0	100 (47/47)	100 (20/20)	100 (47/47)	100 (20/20)
Leber et al.	59[a]	23.7 (14/59)	88 (22/25)	85 (17/20)	88 (22/25)	85 (17/20)
Raff et al.	70	0	95 (38/40)	90 (27/30)	93 (38/41)	93 (27/29)
Mollet et al.	52	1.9 (1/52)	100 (38/38)	92 (12/13)	97 (38/39)	100 (12/12)
Ropers et al.	84	3.6 (3/84)	96 (25/26)	91 (50/55)	83 (25/30)	98 (50/51)
Schuijf et al.	61	1.6 (1/61)	94 (29/31)	97 (28/29)	97 (29/30)	93 (27/29)
Ehara et al.	69	2.9 (2/69)	98 (59/60)	86 (6/7)	98 (59/60)	86 (6/7)
Nikolaou et al.	72	5.6 (4/72)	97 (38/39)	79 (23/29)	86 (38/44)	96 (23/24)
Weustink et al.	77	0	99 (76/77)	87 (20/23)	96 (76/79)	95 (20/21)
Leber et al.	90	2.2 (2/90)	95 (20/21)	90 (60/67)	74 (20/27)	99 (60/61)
Total	701	3.8 (27/701) (95% CI 2.6–5.6)	98 (394/404) (95% CI 95–99)	90 (263/293) (95% CI 86–93]	93 (394/424) (95% CI 90–95)	95 (263/273) (95% CI 93–98)

All values are expressed as per cent with absolute numbers in parentheses.
95% CI, 95% confidence interval; NPV, negative predictive value; PPV, positive predictive value.
[a]Exclusion of patients with stents.

Lesion Severity and Functional Relevance

The limited temporal and spatial resolution of CT may create difficulties in accurately assessing the severity of coronary artery stenoses. There is a tendency to overestimate the degree of luminal narrowing by CT when compared with invasive angiography, and pronounced calcification of a vessel segment can make lesion assessment particularly difficult. Usually, calcification will lead to overestimation, rather than underestimation of lesion severity. Furthermore, CT angiography is limited to anatomic visualization of stenosis rather its functional relevance. (Figure 2) In a head-to-head comparison of MSCCT and nuclear myocardial perfusion imaging with single-photon emission computed tomography (SPECT) in 114 patients with intermediate likelihood of CAD, only 45% of patients with an abnormal MSCCT had an abnormal perfusion on SPECT.

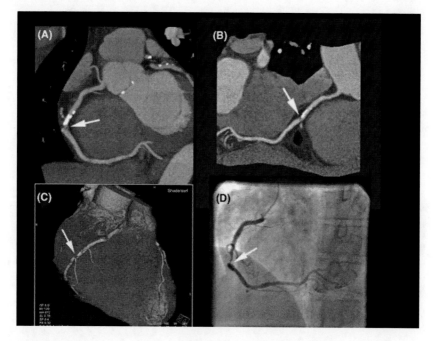

Figure 2. Coronary artery stenosis detection with multi-detector row computed tomography. High-grade stenosis of the mid-right coronary artery in a 55-year-old man with atypical chest pain. (A) A maximum intensity projection, with a high-grade luminal reduction distal to a calcified segment. (B) A curved multi-planar reconstruction. (C) A three-dimensional rendering of the heart and right coronary artery. (D) the corresponding coronary angiogram. (Reproduced with permission).

These findings are in agreement with other preliminary reports which showed that only a fraction of patients with obstructive coronary lesions demonstrate ischemia on SPECT and positron emission tomography (PET) perfusion imaging. This has led to the idea of hybrid imaging to assess the complimentary value of adding functional studies beside anatomical localization. In one study, hybrid PET/CT (Figure 3) was evaluated in patients with suspected CAD, which yielded a sensitivity and specificity of 90 and 98%, respectively, for the detection of hemodynamically relevant coronary lesions. A recent report of a combined CT/SPECT scanner included 56 patients with known or suspected CAD who underwent pharmacologic or exercise stress. All patients underwent invasive coronary angiography within four weeks of the procedure. Compared to the ability of MSCCT to detect stenotic lesions in coronary arteries using x-ray coronary angiography as the gold standard, the use of MSCCT/SPECT to detect hemodynamically significant lesions using x-ray coronary angiography improved sensitivity from 84% to 96% and specificity from 74% to 95%. The predictive values, which will vary between patient populations with differing prevalence of disease, the positive predictive value increased from 61% to 77% and the negative predictive value increased from 90% to 99%.

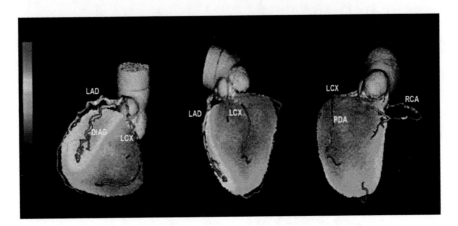

Figure 3. Fused 3D reconstructions of coronary CTA and stress 82Rb myocardial perfusion study obtained in same setting, assessed through integrated PET/CTA. CTA demonstrated 3-vessel CAD. Fused CTA stress myocardial perfusion images demonstrate large area of severe stress-induced perfusion abnormality (deep blue color) only in territory of dominant LCX coronary artery. LAD = left anterior descending coronary artery; DIAG = diagonal artery; LCX = left circumflex coronary artery; RCA = right coronary artery; PDA = posterior descending artery. (Reproduced with permission).

Atherosclerotic Plaque Characterization

MSCCT can be used to assess the calcium score in patients with atherosclerotic coronary artery disease. The dose of radiation used for calcium scoring is 1-2 mSv. While the amount of calcium in an atherosclerotic plaque correlates moderately with the plaque burden, calcification is neither a sign of stability nor instability of individual plaques. In several trials, the absence of coronary calcium ruled out the presence of significant coronary artery stenoses with the negative predictive value of 92-97%. However, even pronounced coronary calcification is not necessarily associated with hemodynamically relevant luminal narrowing. Therefore, even the detection of large amounts of calcium does not indicate the presence of significant stenoses and it should not prompt invasive coronary angiography in otherwise asymptomatic individuals. The major interest in MSCCT is to characterize non-calcified plaques (Figure 4).

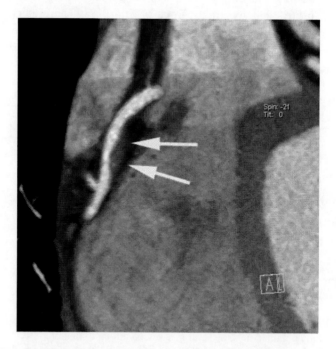

Figure 4. Imaging of coronary atherosclerotic plaque by multidetector row computed tomography. The contrast-enhanced multi-detector row computed tomography data set shows a noncalcified plaque in the proximal right coronary artery with substantial positive remodelling and only a mild associated reduction of the coronary lumen. (Reproduced with permission).

Data on the accuracy of CT angiography to detect non-calcified plaque are limited to a small number of studies that have compared CT angiography with intravascular ultrasound (IVUS). Some data are available concerning plaque characterization by CT. On average, the CT attenuation within 'fibrous' plaques is higher than within 'lipid-rich' plaques (mean attenuation values of 91–116 vs. 47–71 HU) but there is large variability of these measurements, which currently prevents accurate classification of non-calcified 'plaque types' by CT. Motoyama et al, found a significantly higher prevalence of plaque, with a CT attenuation <30 HU in lesions associated with acute coronary syndromes when compared with stable lesions. (Figure 5) Another analysis of 100 patients who were followed for 16 months after coronary CT angiography demonstrated a higher cardiovascular event rate in patients with non-obstructive plaque detected by MSCCT compared with individuals without any plaque. Although these initial observations suggest that there may be a potential value of plaque imaging by CT coronary angiography for risk prediction, one must be aware that reliable visualization of coronary plaque requires the highest possible image quality which goes along with substantial expenses in radiation and contrast agent exposure.

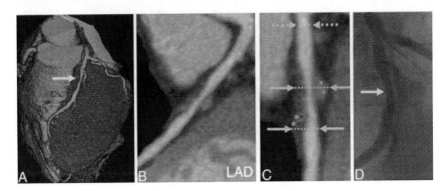

Figure 5. The CT characteristics of a culprit lesion in a 40-year-old male patient presenting with acute coronary syndrome. (A) Volume rendering. (B) Curved MPR. (C) Magnified view of the region of interest from (C). (D) Coronary angiogram. The white arrows in (A) and (D) show the site of luminal obstruction or culprit lesion. As shown by the solid yellow arrows at 2 sites in the culprit lesion in (C), the lesion is positively remodeled as compared with the normal coronary segment proximal to the lesion (denoted by interrupted arrows). Remodeling index in this patient was 1.43. An NCP <30 HU represents the probability of a soft plaque (red circles are placed along the course of low attenuation), and 30 HU <NCP <150 HU denotes a fibrous plaque (green squares). CT = computed tomography; LAD = left anterior descending artery; MPR = multiplanar reformation; NCP = noncalcified plaque (Reproduced with permission).

MSCCT in Acute Coronary Syndrome

There are multiple studies which used MSCCT to triage patients presented with chest pain to rule out acute coronary syndrome (ACS). MSCCT is very valuable in ruling out disease due to its high negative predictive value. Hoffmann et al, evaluated 103 patients who were admitted to the hospital without ischemic ECG changes and/or elevated biomarkers, 64-slice MSCCT was shown to allow accurate triage. Both the absence of coronary plaque and significant coronary stenosis accurately predicted the absence of ACS, with a negative predictive value of 100 %. The positive predictive value was rather low, indicating false-positive results in a considerable number of scans (47% for the detection of significant stenoses, 14/30 positive scans), and only a small percentage of patients with acute chest pain were enrolled in the study (103 of 305 initially screened patients). Another study randomized 197 low-risk acute chest pain patients to either MSCCT or standard diagnostic evaluation. MSCCT allowed immediate diagnosis in 75 percent of patients, while further noninvasive testing was required in 25 percent due to intermediate stenosis severity or non-diagnostic image quality. Nevertheless, MSCCT was faster (3.4 vs 15 hours) in establishing a definitive diagnosis and had a lower cost ($1,586 vs $1,872) compared with the standard of care.

Coronary Stent Imaging

A noninvasive angiographic technique to assess coronary stent patency would be highly desirable. In general, stents are difficult to visualize on MSCCT because of image reconstruction artifacts in the presence of metal. Large caliber (>3 to 3.5 mm) stents in the left main coronary artery, proximal segments of the other coronary arteries (Figure 6) or coronary artery bypass grafts (CABG) have the highest likelihood of being imaged with diagnostic image quality. In a report of 125 stented lesions in 81 patients, the sensitivity and specificity for in-stent restenosis was 91 and 93 percent in evaluable segments (88 percent). In another series of 192 stented lesions in 182 patients, the sensitivity and specificity for in-stent restenosis was 95 and 93 percent in evaluable segments (93 percent) [80]. Only stents ≥ 2.5 mm in diameter were evaluated. Although in carefully selected cases (e.g. large diameter stents in a proximal vessel segment, low and stable heart rate, and absence of excessive image noise) MSCCT may be useful in ruling out in-stent restenosis, routine application of MSCCT to assess patients with coronary stents should be cautious. The use of kernel filter has significantly diminished the amount of blooming artifact caused by the metallic stent struts and recently has evolved a standard for evaluation of patients with prior stents.

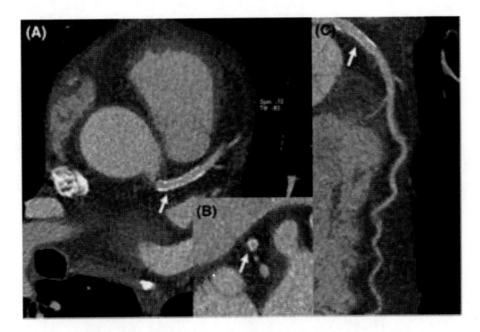

Figure 6. Assessment of coronary artery stents by multi-detector row computed tomography angiography. Example of a stent placed in the proximal part of the left anterior descending coronary artery. Image quality is good and the coronary artery lumen within the stent canbeassessed. multi-detector row computed tomography shows absence of significant in-stent-stenosis. (A) Longitudinal view; (B) axial orientation; (C) curved multiplanar reconstruction.(Reproduced with permission).

Other Coronary Applications of MSCCT

MSCCT can be used for evaluation of patients with prior CABG with high sensitivity and specificity because of the relatively large caliber of the grafts and their relative lack of motion at least in its proximal and mid segments. In comparison, the distal anastomosis can be difficult to assess with confidence because it moves with the coronary artery and its dimensions approximate those of a middle or distal coronary artery segment (ie, ≤ 2 mm). These problems are diminishing with each successive generation of CT scanners. It is also necessary to assess the native coronaries in this subset of patients since myocardial ischemia may result from new lesions in previously un-bypassed vessels or in bypassed vessels distal to the anastomosis. Despite the high diagnostic accuracy of MSCCT for evaluation of coronary grafts, practically most of the patients are referred for invasive coronary angiography regardless of the findings in MSCCT because of the high pretest probability of obstructive CAD in this subset of patients and presence of heavily calcified native vessels, which frequently precludes accurate evaluation.

MSCCT can also be used in patients with known or suspected coronary artery anomalies. It can accurately detect and define the anatomic course of the anomalous coronary arteries and their relation to other cardiac and non-cardiac structures. (Figure 7) It may be even superior to invasive coronary angiography in this matter due to the 3D nature of the data set. Other potential applications of cardiac CTA include evaluation of cardiac allograft vascuopathy, and presence of coronary artery aneurysms in patients with suspected Kawasaki disease.

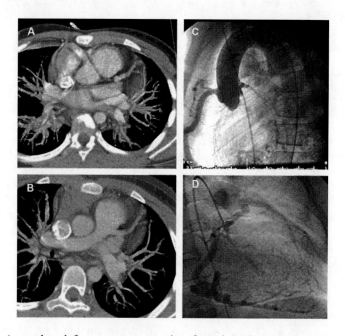

Figure 7. Anomalous left coronary artery arises from the pulmonary artery. (A) & (B) MSCCT reconstructed images (C) Aortogram showing only the right coronary artery coming from the aorta (D) Pulmonary arteriogram showing the origin of the left coronary artery. (Reproduced with permission).

    B. Non coronary application of MSCCT.

Left Atrium and Pulmonary Venous Anatomy

CT imaging allows accurate imaging of the anatomy of both atrial and pulmonary venous return, and in this context, the role of MSCCT in performing electrophysiological procedures such as catheter ablation has rapidly expanded over the past few years. MSCCT can provide a detailed 'roadmap' for these ablation procedures by visualizing the highly variable pulmonary vein anatomy with the use of volume-rendered three-dimensional reconstructions and cross-sectional images (Figure 8). In a series of 201 patients undergoing MSCCT scanning, Marom et al. noted a left-sided 'common ostium' in 14% of the patients and an additional right-sided pulmonary vein in 28% of the patients.

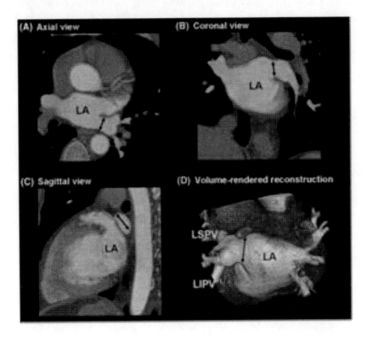

Figure 8. Imaging of the pulmonary veins by multi-detector row computed tomography. Anatomical variation of the pulmonary veins: a single insertion or 'common ostium' of the left-sided pulmonary veins is present. The veins come together before they drain in the left atrium (indicated by the black arrows). This is clearly depicted in the different orthogonal views (A, B, and C) and the volume-rendered reconstruction (D). LA, left atrium; LIPV, left inferior pulmonary vein; LSPV, left superior pulmonary vein. (Reproduced with permission).

By delineating surrounding structures such as the aorta, coronary arteries, and the esophagus, MSCCT is of great value to avoid complications during the ablation procedure. Recently, it has become feasible to integrate the anatomical information derived from MSCCT with the electro-anatomical information from cardiac mapping systems to plan radiofrequency ablation of complex cardiac arrhythmias. These image integration systems allow the use of anatomy derived from MSCCT during the actual ablation procedure (Figure 9). Visualization of the catheter position in relation to the endocardial border, the pulmonary veins, and surrounding structures, performance of catheter ablation procedures may further be facilitated. Initial data indicate that the use of these image integration systems may enhance safety, reduce procedure time, and improve the outcome of ablation procedures for atrial fibrillation. In addition, MSCCT is important in the follow-up for complications of patients after catheter ablation procedures. The use of MSCCT in the identification of pulmonary vein stenosis after catheter ablation has been described extensively and MSCCT is an inherent part in the care of these patients.

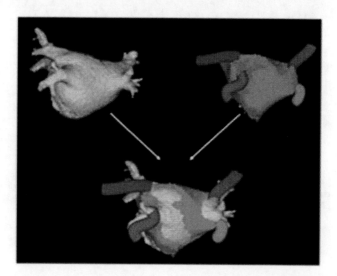

Figure 9. Fusion imaging in electrophysiology using multi-detector row computed tomography and electro-anatomical mapping. Integration of multi-detector row computed tomography and electro-anatomic map for catheter ablation of atrial fibrillation. With the use of image integration systems, the anatomy of the left atrium and pulmonary veins derived from the multi-detector row computed tomography (upper left panel) can be fused with the electroanatomic map (upper right panel). The 'real' anatomy of the left atrium and pulmonary veins can then be used to guide the catheter ablation procedure (lower panel). (Reproduced with permission).

MSCCT and Cardiac Resynchronization Therapy (CRT)

Up to 40 % of patients who receive CRT device do not respond appropriately, researchers have been trying to determine anatomical and/or physiological factors that can predict a better response to CRT. MSCCT has been introduced as the best way to visualize anatomy of the venous system of the heart to guide left ventricular lead placement. Along with other imaging modalities like echocardiography, Cardiac MR, or PET scan, it may help determine the LV lead placement in relation to the scar tissue, however, data on the routine use of MSCCT prior to CRT is scarce and routine use is controversial.

Myocardial Viability and Perfusion

Several pre-clinical and clinical studies have documented that MSCCT allows assessment of myocardial viability by studying 'late enhancement' in a similar fashion as cardiac MR. In the setting of acute, subacute, and chronic occlusive coronary artery disease, myocardial perfusion defects can be observed on the first pass of the contrast bolus ('early defect'). Subsequently in the setting of myocardial infarcts, 5–15 min following contrast infusion, late hyper-enhancement becomes apparent (Figure 10).

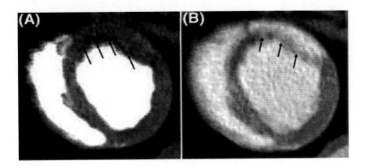

Figure 10. Assessment of perfusion and viability by multidetector row computed tomography. First-pass and delayed enhanced multi-detector row computed tomography myocardial imaging in a porcine model of subacute myocardial infarction. (A) demonstrates an 'early defect' in the anterior wall (arrows) during first-pass of the contrast bolus; (B) demonstrates a hyperenhanced, 'late defect' in the anterior myocardial wall (arrows) imaged 10 min following contrast infusion. (Reproduced with permission).

Furthermore, there is pre-clinical and preliminary clinical evidence that contrast-enhanced MSCCT can provide assessment of myocardial perfusion. As a complement to the morphological information of CT coronary angiography, the assessment of myocardial perfusion might be of clinical utility in assessing hemodynamic significance of an anatomical obstruction. George et al. demonstrated in an animal model of coronary stenosis that MSCCT angiography protocols, when performed during adenosine infusion, can provide semi-quantitative measures of myocardial perfusion.

Congenital Heart Disease

Because of the high spatial and temporal resolution, rapid image acquisition, 3D volume data acquisition, and advanced post-processing tools, MSCCT has become an important non-invasive diagnostic examination both in children and in adults with congenital heart disease. MSCCT is a valuable tool in the pre-operative evaluation of cardiac anomalies (such as tetralogy of Fallot) and the follow-up of baffles and shunts. Patients with untreated patent ductusarteriosus or coarctation of the aorta and those with anomalous pulmonary venous return can also be evaluated accurately with MSCCT. Furthermore, MSCCT can depict coronary artery anatomy, which is often anomalous in patients with congenital heart disease. Cook and Raman evaluated the MSCCT data sets of 85 patients with congenital cardiovascular disease. The relationship of the great vessels, number and location of the coronary ostia, and proximal course of the coronaries could be identified in all cases, and coronary anomalies were detected in 16 of the 85 patients. Despite the fact that MSCCT provides detailed anatomic information, which is of major importance in the care of patients with congenital heart disease, it has to be taken into account that exposure to radiation during follow-up of these patients mainly stems from CT scans and angiography. In particular, when serial evaluation over time is needed, non-ionizing imaging procedures (such as MRI and echocardiography) should be considered. On the other hand, MSCCT scanning is not hampered by the presence of pacemakers and metal artifacts and therefore may be indicated in patients with implanted devices if echocardiography does not provide all clinically necessary information. The utility of CT imaging in patients with congenital heart disease may well extend beyond the heart itself, to include structures such as the pulmonary vessels which are often affected in these patients and may be difficult to evaluate by echocardiography.

Cardiac Computed Tomography Imaging

Risks Associated with MSCCT

Exposure to ionizing radiation from medical imaging may have deterministic as well as stochastic effects. A deterministic effect is one in which severity is determined by the dose. A dose threshold (ie, a dose below which an effect is not seen) is characteristic of a deterministic effect. An example of deterministic effect would be a skin burn that may happen during cardiovascular procedure or imaging. While a stochastic effect represents an outcome for which the probability of occurrence (rather than severity) is determined by the dose. An example is radiation-induced carcinogenesis, which occurs after a typically prolonged but variable delay (latency) after exposure. The main health risk associated with MSCCT use is the stochastic effect.

The radiation sensitivity of biological cells is related to the rate of proliferation, number of future divisions, and degree of differentiation. It is undisputed that ionizing radiation can cause chromosomal changes and that high doses of radiation are associated with an increase in malignancies. However, only some chromosomal changes will translate into phenotypic illness. The carcinogenic potential of ionizing radiation is also affected by the intrinsic, substantial background risk of cancer of the general population and the ubiquity of natural background radiation. Given the many confounding issues, together with the difficulties related to determining patient-specific radiation doses accurately and the latency period of 10 to 40 years for most radiation-induced solid malignancies, studies designed to examine possible carcinogenic effects of ionizing radiation at the levels used in cardiovascular imaging require very large sample sizes and many years of follow-up. These circumstances make it unlikely, if not impossible, to empirically verify the risk of malignancy of low levels of radiation in clinical prospective studies.

The radiation dose during MSCCT is relatively high (5-20 mSv) but still lower than nuclear medicine scans. (Table 3) Great effort has been tried to reduce the amount of radiation during cardiovascular imaging. Reductions in radiation dose can be achieved by obvious and straightforward measures, such as keeping the length of the scan volume and tube current as short and as low as possible. Another effective way of reducing radiation dose is the use of ECG-correlated tube current modulation, in which the full tube current is limited to a short-time period in diastole, resulting in the reduction of radiation dose by 30–40%. Tube current modulation is particularly effective in low heart rates.

Table 3. Representative Values and Ranges of Effective Dose Estimates Reported in the Literature for Selected Radiological Studies (Reproduced with permission)

Examination	Representative Effective Dose Value (mSv)	Range of Reported Effective Dose Values (mSv)	Administered Activity (MBq)
Chest x-ray PA and lateral	0.1	0.05–0.24	NA
CT chest	7	4–18	NA
CT abdominal	8	4–25	NA
CT pelvis	6	3–10	NA
Coronary calcium CT*	3	1–12	NA
Coronary CT angiogram†	16	5–32	NA
64-Slice coronary CTA‡			
Without tube current modulation	15	12–18	NA
With tube current modulation[21]	9	8–18	NA
Dual-source coronary CTA‡			
With tube current modulation	13	6–17	NA
Prospectively triggered coronary CTA‡[22]	3	2–4	NA
Diagnostic invasive coronary angiogram	7	2–16	NA
Percutaneous coronary intervention or radiofrequency ablation	15	7–57	NA
Myocardial perfusion study			
Sestamibi (1-day) stress/rest	9	—	1100
Thallium stress/rest	41	—	185
F-18 FDG	14	—	740
Rubidium-82	5	—	1480

Furthermore, reducing tube voltage to 100 kV instead of the commonly used 120 kV results in a substantial further reduction of radiation exposure and should be considered in patients with a low-to-moderate body mass.

In summary, the radiation dose from cardiac CTA is not low, but is very comparable to other cardiovascular imaging modalities. Although, there is a risk of developing a malignancy from radiation exposure associated with cardiac CTA, it seems to be very low. A recent statement on ionizing radiation in cardiac imaging by the AHA Science Advisory estimated a risk of fatal malignancy or lifetime odds of dying per 1000 individuals associated with a cardiac CTA being 1/6th of the risk associated with average Radon gas exposure in the United States, 1/20th of the risk associated with second hand

Cardiac Computed Tomography Imaging

smoke exposure from a spouse, $1/24^{th}$ of the risk associated with the motor vehicle accident (Table 4).

Table 4. Estimated Risks of Fatal Malignancy or Death Resulting From Radiation Exposure and the Lifetime Odds of Dying as a Result of Selected Activities of Everyday Life
(Reproduced with permission)

Effective radiation dose	
1 mSv (calcium score/lung screen)	0.05
10 mSv (coronary CTA/abdomen CT, invasive coronary angiography, radionuclide myocardial perfusion study)	0.5
50 mSv (yearly radiation worker allowance)	2.5
100 mSv (definition of low exposure)	5
Natural fatal cancer	212
Passive smoking	
Low exposure	4
High exposure, married to a smoker	10
Radon in home	
US average	3
High exposure (1% to 3%)	21
Arsenic in drinking water	
2.5 μg/L (US estimated average)	1
50 μg/L (acceptable limit before 2006)	13
Motor vehicle accident	11.9
Pedestrian accident	1.6
Drowning	0.9
Bicycling	0.2
Lightning strike	0.013

Balancing Benefits and Risks

As a general role, the potential risks of any test must be weighed against the potential benefits of this test. This assessment is difficult when it comes to MSCCT since the health risks related to radiation exposure at the levels common in cardiovascular imaging are controversial. In addition, evidence is limited on the impact of these tests on clinical outcomes. Acknowledging these limitations, an individualized assessment of potential risks and benefits of each imaging procedure is required that incorporates the patient's age and gender, clinical presentation, the health risks implied by the tentative diagnosis for which imaging is to be performed, and the types of imaging modalities that are appropriate to address the clinical question at hand. As an example, MSCCT or radionuclide myocardial perfusion stress testing in a 65-year-old symptomatic man whose chest pain is at intermediate probability of being due to ischemic heart disease, the benefit of identifying treatable, potentially life-threatening coronary artery disease would generally be considered as outweighing the potential risk of imaging associated radiation. In contrast, MSCCT to assess prognosis in an asymptomatic 40-year-old woman by identifying or excluding the presence of subclinical coronary artery plaques ("screening") is not proven to improve quality of life or longevity. In this situation, the potential risk would likely outweigh the potential benefit.

SUMMARY AND CONCLUSION

The most recent generation of MSCCT allows a robust morphological and functional imaging of the heart. Clinically the main focus of MSCCT is coronary artery imaging and since the negative predictive value has been uniformly high, the technique may be the most suitable non-invasive tool to rule out obstructive coronary artery lesions. It is also a valuable and very promising imaging modality in the evaluation of atherosclerotic plaque, coronary artery stents and patients with previous CABG in selected patients. The non-coronary applications of MSCCT are diverse and based mainly on ability of the technique to accurately evaluate the cardiac and vascular anatomy. Finally, the new advances in radiation reduction has made the radiation dose from MSCCT comparable to other cardiovascular imaging procedures which allow for relatively safe scanning without fear of malignant potentials.

REFERENCES

[1] McCollough, C.H. and R.L. Morin, *The technical design and performance of ultrafast computed tomography.* Radiologic clinics of North America, 1994. 32(3): p. 521-36.

[2] Flohr, T.G., et al., *Multi-detector row CT systems and image-reconstruction techniques.* Radiology, 2005. 235(3): p. 756-73.

[3] Kalra, M.K., et al., *Multidetector computed tomography technology: current status and emerging developments.* Journal of computer assisted tomography, 2004. 28 Suppl 1: p. S2-6.

[4] Saini, S., *Multi-detector row CT: principles and practice for abdominal applications.* Radiology, 2004. 233(2): p. 323-7.

[5] Entrikin, D.W., *True high-definition in cardiac imaging will require 4 dimensions of technologic innovation.* Journal of cardiovascular computed tomography, 2009. 3(4): p. 252-6.

[6] Prokop, M., *General principles of MDCT.* European journal of radiology, 2003. 45 Suppl 1: p. S4-10.

[7] Cody, D.D. and M. Mahesh, *AAPM/RSNA physics tutorial for residents: Technologic advances in multidetector CT with a focus on cardiac imaging.*Radiographics : a review publication of the Radiological Society of North America, Inc, 2007. 27(6): p. 1829-37.

[8] Kroft, L.J., A. de Roos, and J. Geleijns, *Artifacts in ECG-synchronized MDCT coronary angiography.* AJR. American journal of roentgenology, 2007. 189(3): p. 581-91.

[9] Schroeder, S., et al., *Cardiac computed tomography: indications, applications, limitations, and training requirements: report of a Writing Group deployed by the Working Group Nuclear Cardiology and Cardiac CT of the European Society of Cardiology and the European Council of Nuclear Cardiology.* European heart journal, 2008. 29(4): p. 531-56.

[10] Leschka, S., et al., *Optimal image reconstruction intervals for non-invasive coronary angiography with 64-slice CT.* European radiology, 2006. 16(9): p. 1964-72.

[11] Leschka, S., et al., *Image quality and reconstruction intervals of dual-source CT coronary angiography: recommendations for ECG-pulsing windowing.* Investigative radiology, 2007. 42(8): p. 543-9.

[12] Wintersperger, B.J., et al., *Image quality, motion artifacts, and reconstruction timing of 64-slice coronary computed tomography angiography with 0.33-second rotation speed.* Investigative radiology, 2006. 41(5): p. 436-42.

[13] Ghostine, S., et al., *Non-invasive detection of coronary artery disease in patients with left bundle branch block using 64-slice computed tomography.* Journal of the American College of Cardiology, 2006. 48(10): p. 1929-34.

[14] Herzog, C., et al., *CT of coronary artery disease.* Journal of thoracic imaging, 2007. 22(1): p. 40-8.

[15] Hoffmann, M.H., et al., *Noninvasive coronary angiography with multislice computed tomography.* JAMA: the journal of the American Medical Association, 2005. 293(20): p. 2471-8.

[16] Leber, A.W., et al., *Quantification of obstructive and nonobstructive coronary lesions by 64-slice computed tomography: a comparative study with quantitative coronary angiography and intravascular ultrasound.* Journal of the American College of Cardiology, 2005. 46(1): p. 147-54.

[17] Raff, G.L., et al., *Diagnostic accuracy of noninvasive coronary angiography using 64-slice spiral computed tomography.* Journal of the American College of Cardiology, 2005. 46(3): p. 552-7.

[18] Heuschmid, M., et al., *ECG-gated 16-MDCT of the coronary arteries: assessment of image quality and accuracy in detecting stenoses.* AJR. American journal of roentgenology, 2005. 184(5): p. 1413-9.

[19] Hoffmann, M.H., et al., *Noninvasive coronary angiography with 16-detector row CT: effect of heart rate.* Radiology, 2005. 234(1): p. 86-97.

[20] Kefer, J., et al., *Head-to-head comparison of three-dimensional navigator-gated magnetic resonance imaging and 16-slice computed tomography to detect coronary artery stenosis in patients.* Journal of the American College of Cardiology, 2005. 46(1): p. 92-100.

[21] !!! INVALID CITATION !!!

[22] Budoff, M.J., et al., *ACCF/AHA clinical competence statement on cardiac imaging with computed tomography and magnetic resonance.* Circulation, 2005. 112(4): p. 598-617.

[23] Ehara, M., et al., *Diagnostic accuracy of 64-slice computed tomography for detecting angiographically significant coronary artery stenosis in an unselected consecutive patient population: comparison with conventional invasive angiography.* Circulation journal : official journal of the Japanese Circulation Society, 2006. 70(5): p. 564-71.

[24] Leber, A.W., et al., *Diagnostic accuracy of dual-source multi-slice CT-coronary angiography in patients with an intermediate pretest likelihood for coronary artery disease.* European heart journal, 2007. 28(19): p. 2354-60.

Cardiac Computed Tomography Imaging

[25] Mollet, N.R., et al., *High-resolution spiral computed tomography coronary angiography in patients referred for diagnostic conventional coronary angiography.* Circulation, 2005. 112(15): p. 2318-23.

[26] Nikolaou, K., et al., *Accuracy of 64-MDCT in the diagnosis of ischemic heart disease.* AJR. American journal of roentgenology, 2006. 187(1): p. 111-7.

[27] Ong, T.K., et al., *Accuracy of 64-row multidetector computed tomography in detecting coronary artery disease in 134 symptomatic patients: influence of calcification.* American heart journal, 2006. 151(6): p. 1323 e1-6.

[28] Ropers, D., et al., *Usefulness of multidetector row spiral computed tomography with 64- x 0.6-mm collimation and 330-ms rotation for the noninvasive detection of significant coronary artery stenoses.* The American journal of cardiology, 2006. 97(3): p. 343-8.

[29] Schuijf, J.D., et al., *Diagnostic accuracy of 64-slice multislice computed tomography in the noninvasive evaluation of significant coronary artery disease.* The American journal of cardiology, 2006. 98(2): p. 145-8.

[30] Weustink, A.C., et al., *Reliable high-speed coronary computed tomography in symptomatic patients.* Journal of the American College of Cardiology, 2007. 50(8): p. 786-94.

[31] Leschka, S., et al., *Accuracy of MSCT coronary angiography with 64-slice technology: first experience.* European heart journal, 2005. 26(15): p. 1482-7.

[32] Budoff, M.J., et al., *Diagnostic performance of 64-multidetector row coronary computed tomographic angiography for evaluation of coronary artery stenosis in individuals without known coronary artery disease: results from the prospective multicenter ACCURACY (Assessment by Coronary Computed Tomographic Angiography of Individuals Undergoing Invasive Coronary Angiography) trial.* Journal of the American College of Cardiology, 2008. 52(21): p. 1724-32.

[33] Miller, J.M., et al., *Diagnostic performance of coronary angiography by 64-row CT.* The New England journal of medicine, 2008. 359(22): p. 2324-36.

[34] Meijboom, W.B., et al., *Diagnostic accuracy of 64-slice computed tomography coronary angiography: a prospective, multicenter, multivendor study.* Journal of the American College of Cardiology, 2008. 52(25): p. 2135-44.

[35] Leschka, S., et al., *Noninvasive coronary angiography with 64-section CT: effect of average heart rate and heart rate variability on image quality.* Radiology, 2006. 241(2): p. 378-85.

[36] Achenbach, S., et al., *Contrast-enhanced coronary artery visualization by dual-source computed tomography--initial experience.* European journal of radiology, 2006. 57(3): p. 331-5.

[37] Scheffel, H., et al., *Accuracy of dual-source CT coronary angiography: First experience in a high pre-test probability population without heart rate control.* European radiology, 2006. 16(12): p. 2739-47.

[38] Schuijf, J.D., et al., *Relationship between noninvasive coronary angiography with multi-slice computed tomography and myocardial perfusion imaging.* Journal of the American College of Cardiology, 2006. 48(12): p. 2508-14.

[39] Gaemperli, O., et al., *Accuracy of 64-slice CT angiography for the detection of functionally relevant coronary stenoses as assessed with myocardial perfusion SPECT.* European journal of nuclear medicine and molecular imaging, 2007. 34(8): p. 1162-71.

[40] Hong, E.C., E.T. Kimura-Hayama, and M.F. Di Carli, *Hybrid cardiac imaging: complementary roles of CT angiography and PET in a patient with a history of radiation therapy.* Journal of nuclear cardiology: official publication of the American Society of Nuclear Cardiology, 2007. 14(4): p. 617-20.

[41] Sampson, U.K., et al., *Diagnostic accuracy of rubidium-82 myocardial perfusion imaging with hybrid positron emission tomography/computed tomography in the detection of coronary artery disease.* Journal of the American College of Cardiology, 2007. 49(10): p. 1052-8.

[42] Namdar, M., et al., *Integrated PET/CT for the assessment of coronary artery disease: a feasibility study.* Journal of nuclear medicine: official publication, Society of Nuclear Medicine, 2005. 46(6): p. 930-5.

[43] Rispler, S., et al., *Integrated single-photon emission computed tomography and computed tomography coronary angiography for the assessment of hemodynamically significant coronary artery lesions.* Journal of the American College of Cardiology, 2007. 49(10): p. 1059-67.

[44] Budoff, M.J., et al., *Assessment of coronary artery disease by cardiac computed tomography: a scientific statement from the American Heart Association Committee on Cardiovascular Imaging and Intervention, Council on Cardiovascular Radiology and Intervention, and Committee*

on *Cardiac Imaging, Council on Clinical Cardiology*. Circulation, 2006. 114(16): p. 1761-91.

[45] Schmermund, A. and R. Erbel, *Unstable coronary plaque and its relation to coronary calcium*. Circulation, 2001. 104(14): p. 1682-7.

[46] Greenland, P., et al., *ACCF/AHA 2007 clinical expert consensus document on coronary artery calcium scoring by computed tomography in global cardiovascular risk assessment and in evaluation of patients with chest pain: a report of the American College of Cardiology Foundation Clinical Expert Consensus Task Force (ACCF/AHA Writing Committee to Update the 2000 Expert Consensus Document on Electron Beam Computed Tomography)*. Circulation, 2007. 115(3): p. 402-26.

[47] Carrascosa, P.M., et al., *Characterization of coronary atherosclerotic plaques by multidetector computed tomography*. The American journal of cardiology, 2006. 97(5): p. 598-602.

[48] Pohle, K., et al., *Characterization of non-calcified coronary atherosclerotic plaque by multi-detector row CT: comparison to IVUS*. Atherosclerosis, 2007. 190(1): p. 174-80.

[49] Schroeder, S., et al., *Non-invasive evaluation of atherosclerosis with contrast enhanced 16 slice spiral computed tomography: results of ex vivo investigations*. Heart, 2004. 90(12): p. 1471-5.

[50] Motoyama, S., et al., *Multislice computed tomographic characteristics of coronary lesions in acute coronary syndromes*. Journal of the American College of Cardiology, 2007. 50(4): p. 319-26.

[51] Pundziute, G., et al., *Prognostic value of multislice computed tomography coronary angiography in patients with known or suspected coronary artery disease*. Journal of the American College of Cardiology, 2007. 49(1): p. 62-70.

[52] Hoffmann, U., et al., *Coronary multidetector computed tomography in the assessment of patients with acute chest pain*. Circulation, 2006. 114(21): p. 2251-60.

[53] Goldstein, J.A., et al., *A randomized controlled trial of multi-slice coronary computed tomography for evaluation of acute chest pain*. Journal of the American College of Cardiology, 2007. 49(8): p. 863-71.

[54] Ligabue, G., et al., *Noninvasive evaluation of coronary artery stents patency after PTCA: role of Multislice Computed Tomography*. La Radiologia medica, 2004. 108(1-2): p. 128-37.

[55] Ehara, M., et al., *Diagnostic accuracy of coronary in-stent restenosis using 64-slice computed tomography: comparison with invasive*

coronary angiography. Journal of the American College of Cardiology, 2007. 49(9): p. 951-9.

[56] Cademartiri, F., et al., *Usefulness of 64-slice multislice computed tomography coronary angiography to assess in-stent restenosis.* Journal of the American College of Cardiology, 2007. 49(22): p. 2204-10.

[57] Ropers, D., et al., *Diagnostic accuracy of noninvasive coronary angiography in patients after bypass surgery using 64-slice spiral computed tomography with 330-ms gantry rotation.* Circulation, 2006. 114(22): p. 2334-41; quiz 2334.

[58] Van de Veire, N.R., et al., *Non-invasive visualization of the cardiac venous system in coronary artery disease patients using 64-slice computed tomography.* Journal of the American College of Cardiology, 2006. 48(9): p. 1832-8.

[59] Jongbloed, M.R., et al., *Multislice computed tomography versus intracardiac echocardiography to evaluate the pulmonary veins before radiofrequency catheter ablation of atrial fibrillation: a head-to-head comparison.* Journal of the American College of Cardiology, 2005. 45(3): p. 343-50.

[60] Jongbloed, M.R., et al., *Atrial fibrillation: multi-detector row CT of pulmonary vein anatomy prior to radiofrequency catheter ablation-- initial experience.* Radiology, 2005. 234(3): p. 702-9.

[61] Marom, E.M., et al., *Variations in pulmonary venous drainage to the left atrium: implications for radiofrequency ablation.* Radiology, 2004. 230(3): p. 824-9.

[62] Tops, L.F., et al., *Fusion of multislice computed tomography imaging with three-dimensional electroanatomic mapping to guide radiofrequency catheter ablation procedures.* Heart rhythm: the official journal of the Heart Rhythm Society, 2005. 2(10): p. 1076-81.

[63] Dong, J., et al., *Integrated electroanatomic mapping with three-dimensional computed tomographic images for real-time guided ablations.* Circulation, 2006. 113(2): p. 186-94.

[64] Burgstahler, C., et al., *Visualization of pulmonary vein stenosis after radio frequency ablation using multi-slice computed tomography: initial clinical experience in 33 patients.* International journal of cardiology, 2005. 102(2): p. 287-91.

[65] Perez-Lugones, A., et al., *Three-dimensional reconstruction of pulmonary veins in patients with atrial fibrillation and controls: morphological characteristics of different veins.* Pacing and clinical electrophysiology: PACE, 2003. 26(1 Pt 1): p. 8-15.

Cardiac Computed Tomography Imaging

107

[66] Piorkowski, C., et al., *Electroanatomic reconstruction of the left atrium, pulmonary veins, and esophagus compared with the "true anatomy" on multislice computed tomography in patients undergoing catheter ablation of atrial fibrillation.* Heart rhythm: the official journal of the Heart Rhythm Society, 2006. 3(3): p. 317-27.

[67] Singh, J.P., et al., *The coronary venous anatomy: a segmental approach to aid cardiac resynchronization therapy.* Journal of the American College of Cardiology, 2005. 46(1): p. 68-74.

[68] Brodoefel, H., et al., *Assessment of myocardial viability in a reperfused porcine model: evaluation of different MSCT contrast protocols in acute and subacute infarct stages in comparison with MRI.* Journal of computer assisted tomography, 2007. 31(2): p. 290-8.

[69] Brodoefel, H., et al., *Sixty-four-MSCT in the characterization of porcine acute and subacute myocardial infarction: determination of transmurality in comparison to magnetic resonance imaging and histopathology.* European journal of radiology, 2007. 62(2): p. 235-46.

[70] Brodoefel, H., et al., *Late myocardial enhancement assessed by 64-MSCT in reperfused porcine myocardial infarction: diagnostic accuracy of low-dose CT protocols in comparison with magnetic resonance imaging.* European radiology, 2007. 17(2): p. 475-83.

[71] Lardo, A.C., et al., *Contrast-enhanced multidetector computed tomography viability imaging after myocardial infarction: characterization of myocyte death, microvascular obstruction, and chronic scar.* Circulation, 2006. 113(3): p. 394-404.

[72] Mahnken, A.H., et al., *Assessment of myocardial viability in reperfused acute myocardial infarction using 16-slice computed tomography in comparison to magnetic resonance imaging.* Journal of the American College of Cardiology, 2005. 45(12): p. 2042-7.

[73] George, R.T., et al., *Multidetector computed tomography myocardial perfusion imaging during adenosine stress.* Journal of the American College of Cardiology, 2006. 48(1): p. 153-60.

[74] Goo, H.W., et al., *Computed tomography for the diagnosis of congenital heart disease in pediatric and adult patients.* The international journal of cardiovascular imaging, 2005. 21(2-3): p. 347-65; discussion 367.

[75] Ou, P., et al., *Three-dimensional CT scanning: a new diagnostic modality in congenital heart disease.* Heart, 2007. 93(8): p. 908-13.

[76] Cook, S.C. and S.V. Raman, *Unique application of multislice computed tomography in adults with congenital heart disease.* International journal of cardiology, 2007. 119(1): p. 101-6.

[77] Hoffmann, A., P. Engelfriet, and B. Mulder, *Radiation exposure during follow-up of adults with congenital heart disease.* International journal of cardiology, 2007. 118(2): p. 151-3.

[78] Gerber, T.C., et al., *Ionizing radiation in cardiac imaging: a science advisory from the American Heart Association Committee on Cardiac Imaging of the Council on Clinical Cardiology and Committee on Cardiovascular Imaging and Intervention of the Council on Cardiovascular Radiology and Intervention.* Circulation, 2009. 119(7): p. 1056-65.

[79] Coles, D.R., et al., *Comparison of radiation doses from multislice computed tomography coronary angiography and conventional diagnostic angiography.* Journal of the American College of Cardiology, 2006. 47(9): p. 1840-5.

[80] Gerber, T.C., et al., *Effect of acquisition technique on radiation dose and image quality in multidetector row computed tomography coronary angiography with submillimeter collimation.* Investigative radiology, 2005. 40(8): p. 556-63.

[81] Einstein, A.J., M.J. Henzlova, and S. Rajagopalan, *Estimating risk of cancer associated with radiation exposure from 64-slice computed tomography coronary angiography.* JAMA: the journal of the American Medical Association, 2007. 298(3): p. 317-23.

[82] Muhlenbruch, G., et al., *Diagnostic value of 64-slice multi-detector row cardiac CTA in symptomatic patients.* European radiology, 2007. 17(3): p. 603-9.

[83] Herzog, P., et al., *[Radiation dose and dose reduction in multidetector row CT (MDCT)].* Der Radiologe, 2002. 42(9): p. 691-6.

[84] Hausleiter, J., et al., *Radiation dose estimates from cardiac multislice computed tomography in daily practice: impact of different scanning protocols on effective dose estimates.* Circulation, 2006. 113(10): p. 1305-10.

In: CT Scans
Editors: V. E. Perkel et al.

ISBN 978-1-62100-319-9
©2012 Nova Science Publishers, Inc.

Chapter 3

NEURODIAGNOSTIC PITFALLS OF CT SCAN FROM NEUROSURGICAL VIEWPOINT: A PERSONAL PERSPECTIVE

Bing H. Tang 唐秉輝

Diplomate, American Board of Neulogical Surgery, 1981 –
Senior Researcher, Research & Ethics, Danville, Calif., U. S.
Scientific Advisor and Research Consultant, Systemic Biology Laboratory,
Institute of Biological Chemistry, Academia Sinica, Taiwan

ABSTRACT

CT scanning, also being called as CAT scanning, is a noninvasive medical test that helps physicians diagnose and treat medical conditions. It combines special x-ray equipment with sophisticated computers to produce multiple images or pictures of the inside of the body. These cross-sectional images of the area being studied can then be examined on a computer monitor, printed or transferred to a compact disc, so-called CD, including internal organs, bones, soft tissue and blood vessels provide greater clarity and reveal more details than regular x-ray exams. Radiologists can more easily diagnose problems such as cancers, cardiovascular disease, infectious disease, appendicitis, trauma and musculoskeletal disorders. It is invaluable in diagnosing and treating spinal problems and injuries to the hands, feet and other skeletal structures because it can clearly show even very small bones as well as surrounding tissues such as muscle and blood vessels. As to the CT scan diagnosis of blood vessel diseases, it is very complex for Central Nervous System. There are diagnostic pitfalls of CT scans in this System.

Methods

1) Reappraisal of Primary Fibrinolytic Syndromes associated with subarachnoid hemorrage, which has been the first report in medical literature since 1973.
2) Analysis and review of Isodensity in CT scans with Bilateral Cerebral Subdural Hematoma
3) Strokes and its Diagnostic Classification
4) Analysis and some review of Cerebral Posterior Circulation Vasculature
5) Analysis of and some reviews on Cocaine use as a Predictor of Nontraumatic SAH
6) Analysis of and some review on Pcom, its rupture, and a different Neurosugical Approach
7) Analysis of some approach to unruptured Aneurysms and AVMs
8) Analysis of ISAT and after ISAT, with a Review of a Clinical Study
9) Analysis and some review of Compression of PoteriorCraneal Fossa
10) Analysis and somereview of Thalamic, Midbrain and Pontine Hemorrage/Infarct
12) Analysis and some review on Vesticular Schwannoma
13) Analysis and review of a case of Hemangiopericytoma
14) Analysis and some review on Children's Sciwora Syndrome

Result

As per aforementioned each section, they are demonstrated and presented respectively.

Conclusion

PrimaryFibrinolytic Syndrome Assocoiated with Subarachniod Hemorrageth at thi author, with two co-authors, reported in 1973, as well, the midbrain and thalamicinfarcts associated with subarachnoid hemorrhage reported were arising from the rupture of a posterior communicating artery aneurysm. [1]

Cerebral Vertebrobasilar System Circulation is confirmed. The so-called 'polar artery' is a synonym of the posterior communicating artery, in which the location of this artery is the similar site of the rupture of an aneurysm reported elsewhere by this author, despite of any possible neurodiagnostic pitfalls of CT scans, which are to be lucidly illustrated as various sections.

In each ensuing related sections of this chapter, whenever possible, neurolosurgical and clinicopathological correlate are suggested.

ABBREVIATIONS

CI confidence interval
CSF Cerebral Spinal Fluid
CT computerized tomography;
FDP Fibrin Degradation Products,
DIC Disseminated Coagulation,
GCS Glasgow Coma Score,
GOS Glasgow Outcome Scale,
HCT Hematocrit,
PLT Platelet, PT Prothrombin Time,
PTT Partial Thromboplastin Time,
INR International Normalized Ratio,
EDH Epidural Hematoma,
SDH Subdural Hematoma,
ICH Intracranial Hemorrhage,
IVH Intraventricular Hemorrhage,
MABP Mean arterial blood pressure,
SAH Subarachnoid Hemorrhage

INTRODUCTION

CT scanning, also being called as CAT scanning, is a noninvasive medical test that helps physicians diagnose and treat medical conditions. It combines special x-ray equipment with sophisticated computers to produce multiple images or pictures of the inside of the body. These cross-sectional images of the area being studied can then be examined on a computer monitor, printed or transferred to a CD. CT scans of internal organs, bones, soft tissue and blood vessels provide greater clarity and reveal more details than regular x-ray exams. Radiologists can more easily diagnose problems such as cancers, cardiovascular disease, infectious disease, appendicitis, trauma and musculoskeletal disorders. It is invaluable in diagnosing and treating spinal problems and injuries to the hands, feet and other skeletal structures because it can clearly show even very small bones as well as surrounding tissues such as muscle and blood vessels. As to CT scan diagnosis of blood vessel diseases, it is very complex for Central Nervous System. Especially when this system is encountering SAH, there are diagnostic pitfalls of CT scans in this System. Those pitfalls are to be discussed and assessed respectively in the following sections.

SECTION 1. REAPPRAISAL OF PRIMARYFIBRINOLYTIC SYNDROMES ASSOCIATED WITH SUBARACHNOID HEMORRAGE

In medical literature, Primary Fibrinolytic Syndromes associated with subarachnoid hemorrhage has been reported since 1973.

Revisiting to an original paper published in Angiology, November, 1973 [1], this author, as the first author, with two coauthors reported the findings of a patient with marked increasing in systemic fibrinolytic activity associated with systemic bleedingfrom a ruptured intracranial aneurysm. This association had not previously been reported prior to 1973.

The probable hypothesis to explain the fibrinolytic syndrome is as following:

- Primary Fibrinolytic Syndrome Associated with Subarachnoid Hemorrhage

Neurodiagnostic Pitfalls of CT Scan from Neurosurgical Viewpoint   113

First Admission

A 62-year-old Caucasian woman, was admitted to a Medical Center of New York City on July 12,1972, with a one-month history of headache, stiffness and pain in the neck, bilateral buttock and right leg pain, difficulty in walking and double vision. The MABP was 154/90 mmHg. There were no outstanding physical or neurologicalfindings. Lumbar puncture was carried out, which revealed cerebrospinal fluid pressures were normal initially, the second CSF was xanthochroid with protein of 80 mg%. The subsequentluid was clear.

Second Admission of the Same Patient

On September 13, 1972, the patient was brought to Hospital in a leghargic state, having been found lying on the floor of her apartment for an undetermined length of time. She was confused, disoriented, dehydrated, and only able to respond to simple commands. Blood pressure was 130/90 mm Hg. Positive physical findings were several small areas of ecchymosis over the right leg, and a third degree burn, sized 5x3 cm over the right lateral thigh. Neurological examination revealed bilateral papilledema with a peripapillary fundal hemorrhage on the right, nuchal rigidity, right hemiparesis, and a dilated right pupil were noted. Both pupils reacted to light.

Laboratory findings revealed decreased platelets, anisocytosis and ecchinocytosis of red blood cells as well as a shift to the left, and toxic granulation of the neutrophils were noted on the peripheral blood smear. Urea nitrogen was 180 mg%, and sodium 121 meq/L. Cerebrospinal fluid (CSF) pressure was 220 mm of CSF. The fluid appeared xanthochromic with protein of 180 mg%, red blood count of 1000 per mm^3 and no white blood cells found.

The initial studies of hemostatic function included following: activated PPT partial thromboplastin time (36 seconds – control 35 seconds);   PT prothrombin time (21 seconds—control 11 seconds);   thrombin time (30 seconds—control 20 seconds); stypven time (21 seconds—control 20 seconds); euglobulinlysis time (35 minutes—control more than 90 minutes); fibrin plate lysis (118 mm^2--control 50mm^2); FDP   fibrinogen degradation products (60ug/ml.—control 16 ug/ml.) and fibrinogen (90mg%--normal 150-350 mg%).

The left carotid and right vertebral angiograms via femoral catheter revealed multiple areas of narrowing of cerebral vessels secondary to spasm.

The narrowing of the cerebral vessels was most prominent over the proximal portions of anterior and middle cerebral arteries of the left side. Severe CE, ICH, IVH, and spasm of the left vertebral artery was noted and this vessel was only filled by the right subclavian route. A small aneurysm was seen in the region of the left posterior communicating artery.

One hour later, after the patient being returned to the ward, the patient was found to be flaccid, unresponsive, diaphoretic and ashen. Her blood pressure at that time, MABP was 70/40 mm Hg and pulse rate was70 per minute. Generalized ecchymosis of the skin was present and there was marked swelling and ecchymosis over the left femoral region at the site of the retrograde femoral catheterization. The patient was treated with steroids, blood transfusion, plasma, epsilon aminocaproic acid and vitamin K1, but she remained comatose and expired twenty four hours after the second dmission.

Post-Mortem Examination

At post-mortem examination, the significant gross findings included: (a) a small ruptured aneurysm of the left posterior communicating artery with extensive hemorrhage into the subarachnoid space. The lumen of the residual aneurismal sac was filled with firmly adherent clotted blood (b) diffuse swelling of the left cerebral hemisphere; (c) a hematoma extending from the region of the left femoral artery to the abdominal wall and retropubic space; (d) three hundred ml. of unclotted blood in the peritoneal cavity; and (e) extensive hemorrhage and ecchymosis of skin, mucous membranes, pericardium, perirenal and perigastric tissue.

Microscopic Finding

Notable microscopic findings were: (a) an aneurysm of the left posterior communicating artery with residual thrombus. The thrombus showed advanced organization at the periphery but no organization centrally; (b) cellular bone marrow revealed with normal erythroid and myeloid tissue but there was absence of megakaryocytes; and (c) no evidence of peripheral vascular thrombi nor arteriolar fibrin deposition. Neither the renal arterioles nor the renal glomeruli showed any fibrin deposition.

Interim Discussion

This patient had at least two episodes of subarachnoid hemorrhage from a ruptured aneurysm of the left posterior communicating artery over a two-month period. The second episode of subarachnoid bleeding was complicated by defective hemostasis due to increased systemic fibrinolysis. Despite the theoretical possibility of increased systemic fibrinolytic activity associated with subarachnoid bleeding, there are no previous reports of such an occurrence in the literature.

In retrospect, there seemed to be two separate events that influenced the increased fibrinolytic activity in this patient. The initial event was most likely connected in some way with the rupture of an aneurysm and subsequent subarachnoid hemorrhage. The second event was related to the performance of the cerebral angiogram cathe3terization.

Fibrinolysis in man is an important homeostatic process [2 - 11] and serves primarily to limit fribrin deposition. Fibrinolysis is mediated by plasmin. Two categories of tissue activators have also been identified an activator present in endothelial cells of blood vessels, and an activator present in the lysosomal granules of cells obtained from a variety of tissue. Of particular significance in this case is the observation of Moltke [3], that large quantities of plasminogen activator are present in the leptomeninges of brain.

Fibronolytic disorders may result from either primary activation of the fibrinolytic system or by secondary activation of this system as a consequence of intravascular coagulation.

Secondary fibrinolytic disorders are found in association with disseminated intravascular coagulation (DIC), an intermediate phase of a wide variety of diseases [12-15]. In intravascular cogulation, the generation of thrombin activities plasminogen. Previous reference was made to the findings of Moltke [3] who demonstrated large amounts of plasminogen activators in the leptomeninges of the brain. It is possible that either the inflammatory reaction caused by blood in the subarachnoid space or ischemia, caused by the subarachnoid hemorrhage, might have initiated the release of plasminogen activators from the leptomeninges and stimulated plasmin formation.

The observation that neuroradiological procedures such as pneumoencephalography in the 1970's, ventriculography and cerebral angiography increased systemic fibrinolysiscerebral angiography increased systemic fibrinolysis was previously reported by Schneck and von Kaulla [16, 17]. The relationship between contrast radiographic studies and systemic fibrinolysis is not entirely clear, but these diagnostic manipulations may at

116   Bing H. Tang

times be associated with transient ischemia of the cerebral circulation. Cerebral ischcmia in turn has been noted to cause the release of tissue activator for plasminogen [18-21].

Key points

Second admission due to rebleeding from aneurysm.Physical examination is important:

- Areas of Ecchymosis.
- The initial studies of hemostatic function is essential.
- The increased fibrinolytic activity also influenced by cerebral angiongram: Marked Ecchymosis over femoral catheterization site.
- Lack of production of platelets (PLT), evidenced by the absence of megakaryocytes.
- No evidence of peripheral vascular thrombi nor arteriolar fibrin deposition, no evidence for DIC.
- Primary fibrinolytic disorder to be kept in the mind as a differential diagnosis.

SECTION 2. A 74-YEAR-OLD MALE: A CASE REPORT IN 1998

The patient, a 74 years old Taiwanese male fell down from the motor vehicle accident on 6, 11, 1998, complained of headache, dizziness and left sided weakness. CT scan was done on August, 11, 1998 at a regional teaching hospital in Mid-Taiwan. It revealed a right sided subdural hematoma, Glascow Coma Scale (GCS): E4V5M4 = 13. 8, 14, 1998 Right parietal chronic and subacute subdural hematoma 150 ml, with subdural membrane were removed. Post-operatively, the patient was doing very well; he removed endotracheeal tube, NG tube and arterial line by himself. His left hemiparesis improved.

On August 22, 1998, post-operative 7th day, the patient vomited three times, he was found was lethargic but arousals, GCS was E3V3M3. His previous left hemiparesis got worse. Neurological examination revealed that

NeurodiagnosticPitfalls of CT Scan from Neurosurgical Viewpoint   117

left Basbinski sign was positive. He had his right arm with ecchymosis sized 23 x 5 cm.

On the same day, the gastric content from his nasogastric tube suction showed that occult blood was positive. Cerebral CT scan revealed that right frontotemporal acute subdural hematoma, which was latter removed in the amount of 15 ml. At that juncture, the CT scan finding appeared to be uneventful, which was straightforward without any pitfalls as far as its interpretation concerned.

Laboratory finding at that juncture revealed as following:

- The HCT count was decreased.
- Prothrombin time (PT) 16.6 (12-16), and partial thrombin time (PTT) 31.6 (24-40), both tests were normal.
- PLT counts were carried out on August 22, 1998, which showed a decreasing from 120,000 to 103,000 mm3; on the following day, it further dropped to 103, 000, and finally decreased to 101,000.
- C Reative Protein test revealed 8.2 mg/L on August 13, 1998 (The normal value should be less than 0.8 mg/L; normal CRP values vary from lab to lab. Generally, there is no C Reative Protein detectable in blood.)

Also due to ecchymotic areas were over the patient's bilateral arms and legs, right forearm (with petechiae), chest, and back; under the clinical impression of DIC, the patient was then transferred to a Mid-Taiwan medical center for further haematological management. [2]

SECTION 3. PONDAAG'S REPORT IN 1979

Pondaag in 1979 reported that in 46 head-injured patients coagulation studies were performed immediately after admission. In 76% of all cases signs of disseminated intravascular coagulation (DIC) were found. [21] DIC was related to the severity of the injury and outcome. It is suggested that DIC may be used as an important parameter in assessing craniocerebral trauma. [22]

Pondaag et al.explored in more details the relationship between outcome after head-injury and signs of DIC, as detected by laboratory studies performed in the first few hours after injury. [22]

Very interestingly, Greenberg, Cohen and Cooper in 1985 reported 13 patients with acute subdural and epidural hematomas were found to have fresh, unclotted blood at the time of surgical decompression several hours after injury. Computed tomographic (CT) scans' diagnostic pitfalls of these patients demonstrated areas of hyperdensity, corresponding to clotted hematoma, admixed with areas of isodensity, corresponding to liquid blood. Active bleeding from identifiable loci was found in 11 patients, 4 of them had massive haemorrhages. [23]

Indeed, active bleeding from identifiable loci contributes to impaired hemostasls and spontaneous hemorrhage as DIC occurs in 30-56% of patients who have head trauma [3, 4], and its presence is a significant risk factor for death [3].

Nonetheless, special features of another case reported by Boyko et al.[24] is the isodense nature of an acute subdural hematoma seen on head CT only with contrast enhancement. Such an isodense, or liquid hematoma would require the almost total absence of clot. [24]. In most experience, this state of affairs is uncommon in DIC, but could indicate active or recurrent hemonhage [4]. More probably, the patient described by Boyko had an unusually severe consumption of his fibrinogen (the level was <10 mg/dl) or underlying hypofibrinogenemia from liver disease or both. Nonetheless, the Boyko et al's use of contrast enhancement was important in this case for the evaluation of an otherwise unexplained midline shift.

Alternatively, subdural hematoma from DIC might have been suspected if the patient had had purpura, easy bruisatillty, and bleeding from vessel puncture sites.

Key points

- DIC is related to the severity if head injury/subarachnoid hemorrhage, including EDH.
- DIC may be used as an important parameter in assessing head trauma.
- DIC is associated with a more severe grade of head trauma and an increased mortality.
- Be careful when Isodensity seen in CT of brains.

"Hyperacute" lesions of CT is generally indicating the following two possibilities:

1) Ongoing active intracranial bleeding, or
2) An onset of coagulopathy [22]

- Be watchful for the management when head trauma / subarachnoid hemorrhage associated with coagulopathy.
- Be alert if the patients have ecchymosis, purpura, easy bruisatility, and bleeding from intravenous or catheter sites.

SECTION 4. STROKE AND ITS DIAGNOSTIC CLASSIFICATION

Next to coronary heart disease and cancer, apoplectic insult is the third major cause of death in both the U S and Germany. [25] Due to lack of efficient treatment concepts in conventional medicine, strokes are the most common cause of invalidity in old age. Approximately, twenty percent of those affected expired immediately as a result.

As far as the diagnostic classification of strokes concerned, this author feels that there has been never an existence of any other classification, which would be better than a classification as following from the New York City Neurological Institutefrom from 1973 to 1974 :

(After Neurological Institute in New York City 1973-1974)

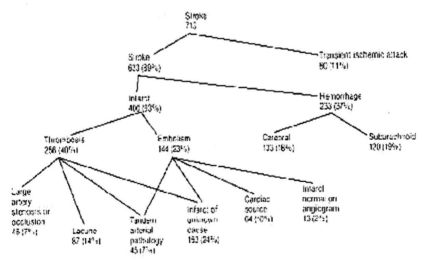

SECTION 5. POSTERIOR COMMUNICATING ARTERY ANEURYSMS AND ITS RUPTURE: NEUROSURGICAL TECHNICAL PITFALLS

The posterior communicating artery aneurysms correspond on 25% of all ruptured aneurysms. The clinical course is typically a subarachnoid hemorrhage and third nerve palsy [1] (Weber's syndrome as another case report will be introduced vide infra.).

Php de Aguiar et al.last year (2010) introduced a new classification for posterior communicating artery aneurysms aneurysms to assist neurosurgeons in daily practice. They also reviewed their experience in posterior communicating artery aneurysms and discussed the major attributing factors affecting morbidity, mortality, symptomatology, and prognosis of these aneurysms. [26]

Noticeably, de Aguiar et al.reviewed historical records, images, craniotomy videos, and CDs of totally 46 surgically clipped aneurysms in their 39 patients from June 2000 to July 2009, in two different Institutions: Hospital São Camilo and Santa Paula, São Paulo, Brazil. Those clipped aneurysms were categorized in two groups, the A group composed by patients who presented clinical subarachnoid hemorrhage in acute stage, while the B group composed by incidental aneurysms carriers. All patients were categorized according to Hunt-Hess scale. (27, 28)

For the aim of helping the general readership's convenience in referring to, Hunt-Hess scale is defined as following:

For Non-Traumatic Sub-Arachnoid Hemorrhage Patients

Description Grade:

- Asymptomatic, mild headache, slight nuchal rigidity 1
- Moderate to severe headache, nuchal rigidity, no neurologic deficit other than cranial nerve palsy 2
- Drowsiness / confusion, mild focal neurologic deficit 3
- Stupor, moderate-severe hemiparesis 4
- Coma, decerebrate posturing 5[27, 28]

Neurodiagnostic Pitfalls of CT Scan from Neurosurgical Viewpoint   121

PhP de Aguiar et al's review can be tabulated for an easy glance as following:

Table 1. PhP de Aguiar et al.'s review can be tabulized for readers' convenience as following

Age	The average age of the patient discovered by them was 53.6 years old (minimum 28 to Maximum 92).
The Prevalence	was higher among women (3.6:1).
The mortality rate	was 20% in group A and none was found in group B. Similar rate was discovered for rupture cases (20% in A group versus zero in B group).
The Aneurysmal size	The mean aneurismal size for A group was 6 mm (ranging from 5 to 25 mm) and 5.3 mm (ranging from 3 to 10 mm) for B group

Thus, the authors noted that posterior communicating artery aneurysms took place 3 to 4 times more frequently in women than man. Oculomotor palsy associated with severe headache, just as showed in this author et al' reported case in 1973 [1], has been commonly related to posterior circulation artery aneurysms. Type II aneurysms (temporal) were indeed the most frequently discovered in PhP de Aguiar et al's review. [26] On the other hand, the worst prognosis in cases with acute hemorrahge took place with fatal variant circulation. Intratentorial aneurysms, basically those with increased degrade using Hunt-Hess criteria (27, 28), have the worst prognosis. In contrary, infundibular aneurysms had the best outcomes with surgical clipping. [26]

SECTION 6. DIFFERENT APPROACH FOR NEUROSURGICALLY EXPROLING POTERIOR COMMUNICATING ARTERY ANEURYSMS

As contrast to what used to be conventional pterional approach, Tetsuyoshi Horiuchi et al.have proposed anterior subtemporal approach for the posterior communicating artery aneurysm protruding posteriorly [29]. They reported their experience with the anterior subtemporal approach for the posterior communicating artery aneurysm protruding posteriorly. Between

2000 and 2005, seven patients with posterior communicating artery aneurysm were operated on through the anterior subtemporal approach. The approach provided a better view than the pterional approach. This new approach appears to be suitable for posteriorly projecting posterior communicating artery aneurysms. The benefits of the anterior subtemporal approach may be tabulated according to their research and clinical experience as following:

Table 2. Tetsuyoshi Horiuchi et al's anterior subtemporal approach for the posterior communicating artery aneurysm [29]

Tetsuyoshi Horiuchi et al's anterior subtemporal approach for the posterior communicating artery aneurysm protruding posteriorly [29]	(1) It provides a short and a direct trajectory to the aneurysm.
	(2) Aneurysmal neck and surrounding structures can be easily identified and secured compared with the pterional approach. .
	(3.) A previously placed clip for a middle cerebral artery or internal carotid artery aneurysm through the pterional route does not interfere with the clipping surgery for regrown or de novo posterior communicating artery aneurysms

SECTION 7. ONE OF THE PREDICATORS OF SUBARACHNOID HEMORRAGE

It is interesting to note that intranasal cocaine is, as well, used commonly as a local anesthetic during many rhinolaryngologic procedures. Although its "recreational" use in high doses (such as what have been reported in Howington et al's study. [33] Most of the 36 patients in their study have been associated with chest pain and myocardial infarction. Such an association has not been well established when cocaine is used in low doses as a topical anesthetic; more over, its effect on the coronary vasculature of humans is still unknown. Lange et al.[34] investigated the effects of intranasal cocaine (10 percent cocaine hydrochloride; 2 mg per kilogram of body weight) of the blood flow, and found on myocardial oxygen demand in 45 patients (34 men and 11 women, 36 to 67 years of age) who were undergoing cardiac catheterization for the evaluation of chest pain. Lange et al.concluded that the intranasal administration of cocaine near the dose used for topical anesthesia causes vasoconstriction of the coronary arteries, with a decrease in the coronary blood flow, in spite of an increase in myocardial oxygen demand, and that these effects are arbitrated by alpha-adrenergic stimulation. It is then reasonable to assume that these effects would be more pronounced at the much higher doses associated with the recreational use of cocaine such as what was used in the study by Howington and his coworkers. [33] Hence, this author (Tang, B) agrees with Howington et al's suggestion to recognize cocaine-use as a major systemic disease when determining Hunt and Hess grading for the classification of aneurismal subarachnoid hemorrhage. [27, 28, 35]

Nonetheless, in their study, Howington et al. agree that the higher percentage of Fisher Grade 3 hemorrhages [36] seen in the cocaine user group of their study was not statistically significant, they believe that the results suggest an association between cocaine use and an increase in the amount of subarachnoid blood on clinical manifestation. The results of their study have well demonstrated that cocaine adversely affects Hunt and Hess grade, independent of the effect of cocaine *per se* on MABP.

In Howington et al's study, the authors present the result of influence of increased amount of hemorrhage at the time of aneurismal rupture, as measured using the Fisher grade, extends beyond the initial clinical presentation. As the amount of blood in the subarachnoid space increases so does the risk of vasospasm. 1)The indirect exacerbation of post-SAH vasospasm is coupled with the fact that cocaine use has also been shown to cause cerebrovascular spasm directly. [33, 35] The association between cocaine use and negative outcome in patients with SAH has long been connected to the effect of the drug *per se* on the patient. [7, 9, 33, 35] This indirect association already has its own existence; nonetheless, Howington et al's study has definitely made additional suggestion of a direct correlation between cocaine use and the authors' own patient population. [7, 9, 33]

With regard to the effect of cocaine to the increase of amount of subarachnoid blood, noticeably, Fisher CM and his coworker's work of 'Relation of cerebral vasospasm to subarachnoid hemorrhage' appears to be able to visualize the size of subarachnoidal blood clot via CT scanning, despite of whatsoever diagnostic pitfalls of CT scans involved. [11, 33]

As the grading system used at that time (Fisher's article was published in 1980) is partly subjective, the findings based on Fisher's grading system should be regarded as preliminary at that juncture.[36] The result, if confirmed, indicates that blood localized in the subarachnoid space in enough amounts at specific sites is the only important etiological feature in vasospasm-formation. It should be possible to identify patients in danger from vasospasm and then organize early preventive measures. [36 ====== 43

Since cocaine-use has such a negative effect on the management of aneurismal SAH, it appears to be reasonable to suggest that one should consider cocaine-use equal to the presence of a major systemic illness when applying Hunt and Hess grade and predicting clinical outcome.

SECTION 8. UNRUPTURED ANEURYSMS AND/OR UNRUPTURED ARTERIAL VENOUS MALFORMATION (AVM)

As to Unruptured Aneurysms and/or Arterial Venous Malformation, general speaking, the aim of treatment in an unruptured aneurysm/AVM is not to prevent early rebleeding, which we know endovascular therapy is very effective in achieving such a goal, but to a certain extent to heal the aneurysm enduringly and prevent upcoming bleeding, for which we alll know that open microsurgery attains very successful result.

Noticeably, as a recent clinical research example, there is a clinical trial entitled a Trial on endovascular treatment of unruptured intracranial aneurysms (TEAM) [44]. In fact, this intervention is not a crossover trial because it concerns non-compliant case-crossover. It is merely a 'case crossover' (i.e. patients switch from the intended therapy to an alternative therapy). It can thus be observed that non-compliant crossover intervention is not a crossover trial despite the fact that the word of 'crossover' is mentioned. After reaching and then understanding the proposal of the unruptured aneurismal (TEAM) study [44], it obviously indicates that it indeed is not a crossover trial. [45 Altman]

The term of CROSSOVER being used HERE in the aforementioned article is merely in a concept that is applied for 'a phenomenon' occurring in serious disease, e.g. aneurysms, whereby patient's failure leads to switch in therapy. [46, 47] Or it is for the phenomenon that may be studied in connection with non-compliance in clinical trials whereby patients 'cross over'

Neurodiagnostic Pitfalls of CT Scan from Neurosurgical Viewpoint   125

in an unplanned way from one treatment to another. Generally speaking, the specific crossover from the conservative (medical) treatment arm to the surgical arm is well defined as a part of the trial. Such a study requires achievement of sensitive as well as specific endpoints (or a fixed period of time). With regard to discussion of real definition of '*endpoint*', readers are to be referred to one of this author's other articles. (48, Tang B, 2008)

Nonetheless, the main paragraph of that proposal of TEAM [44] is as following:

"The Principal Investor and executive group are committed to verbalizing the equipoise principle innumerable times at workshops, with bulletins, and direct communications to remind participants the reasons for the trial. It is recognized that few crossovers, ideally none, can be tolerated. In all centres, collaborators will provide a compassionate, competent, available environment to rapidly see patients when concerns arise and to provide reassurance when appropriate. Until evidence shows one treatment is best, dissuasion of crossover is ethical. We admit that treatment of a subject allocated to observation, after repeated visits to the emergency room with severe headaches, may constitute an appropriate response, from a medical or moral point of view, and as such is considered an integral aspect of 'conservative management'. We may have to accept some crossovers, but every instance will be vigorously challenged. Crossovers will be followed in their assigned group for intention to treat analyses, but they will be flagged for secondary analyses. The proposed trial carries some analogy with a trial on endarterectomy for asymptomatic carotid stenosis (ACST). Compliance to group assignment was reported to be 95%." [44]

That discussed, with regard to asymptomatic severe carotid artery narrowing or even (ACSC), DOPPLER scan can never be an excellent neurodiagnostic procedure for it. Nevertheless, this author had a male patient who was only 43 years old was diagnosed with ACSC based on an incidental finding of the following Doppler procedure:

CEREBROVASCULAR EVALUATION

AGE 43   SEX M

PERIORBITAL ARTERY DOPPLER
MEDASONICS D10 8 HZ PROBE

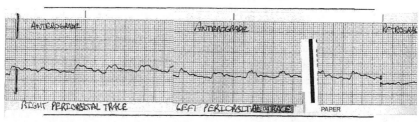

NORMAL ANTEROGRADE FLOW ✓   NORMAL ANTEROGRADE FLOW ✓
ABNORMAL RETROGRADE FLOW ___   ABNORMAL RETROGRADE FLOW ___

CAROTID PULSE TRACINGS
MEDASONICS D10 5HZ PROBE

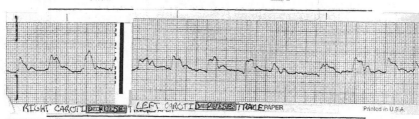

Neurodiagnostic Pitfalls of CT Scan from Neurosurgical Viewpoint

HIGH RESOLUTION REAL-TIME B-MODE CAROTID ARTERY SONOGRAM
HIGH-STOY SP100-B SMALL PARTS SCANNER

RIGHT   LEFT

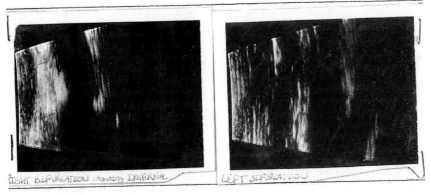

COMMENT:

    RIGHT SIDE: Large plaques on the anterior and posterior walls of the right internal just above the bifurcation.

    LEFT SIDE: No pathology is detected ultrasonically.

SECTION 9. ISAT AND VASCULAR NEUROSURGERY SINCE ISAT

An article with its title as 'Vascular Neurosurgery since the International Subarachnoid Aneurysm Trial' is an interesting one. It raises an important issue of patients whether they should be treated Endovascularly or Neurosurgically?' This article was written by Crocker et al. [48]

This author, Tang, read with interest Crocker el al's paper entitled "Subarachnoid Aneurysm Trial (ISAT) era" in the United Kingdom.

It will certainly be useful to design a clinical study where those patients randomized to the control group could cross over to the interventional group after some pre-defined period of time or after meeting some sort of reasonable endpoint. With respect to endpoints, there appear to have proper concepts involved. An "endpoint" does not mean the "measure" or "severity" of diseases alone, at least to this author (Tang). There are, indeed, different end points in certain diseases, hence we ought to combine them and improve the informational content of categorical clinical trial end points. It is a valuable experience in the U K that can certainly be referred into a more general and specifically a U S perspective. Some opinions mentioned in that article are worthy for our reflection. At the outset, data analysis of Crocker el al's study revealed that a predominant role for endovascular management for acute rupture (86.6 vs 13.4%) of intracraneal cerebral aneurysm, with an inch by inch greater position for open type microsurgery in the more non-compulsory background (57% endovascular vs 43% surgical). They, in addition, reviewed 66 interventions for arteriovenous malformations (AVM), of which merely 6 were surgical. These information are in contrast against a sample year from 2001 to 2002 (pre-International Subarachnoid Aneurysm Trial), viewing as good as rates of surgically treated aneurysms as related to endovascularly treated aneurysms, nonetheless, an increasing entirely in the number of patients requiring open microneurosurgery. The authors realized that exceptional results for microsurgical clipping compared with endovascular therapy could hence be obtained within the current ambiance. These and previously reported studies profoundly establish a ongoing position for vascular neurosurgery as a subspecialist interest in collaboration with a professional endovascular service and a multidisciplinary squad, which is counting but not limited to neuroradiology and neuroanesthesia. [48]

That being reviewed and then assessed, it would be functional to propose a clinical study where those randomized to the control group could cross over to the interventional group subsequent to some pre-defined period of time or after meeting some sort of reasonable endpoint. With respect to endpoints, there appear to have proper concepts involved. An "endpoint" does not denote the "measure" or "severity" of diseases on it own, at least to this author. There are certainly different end points in certain diseases, hence we are supposed to combine them and improve the informational content of categorical clinical trial end points. [49]

The amount of time and the endpoint would need to be tailored to the particular disease - intracraneal aneurysms or AVM or even both, regardless of whether the patients are to be treated in the radiology department or in the Operating Room.

At this juncture of discussion, it is worthwhile to note about what is the real definition of an endpoint? After all, it appears to be a very hilarious thing about neuroscience writing is that one word might fit perfectly – *endpoint* is one along with *capricious* is another. For example, the latter describe, neuropathologically, how a Golgi stain permeates some neurons perfectly and completely, while others remained unstained. In fact, *capricious* is really not appropriate in a biochemical sense, as the term means 'at random'. Nevertheless, outside of biochemistry and neuropathology, *capricious* has a connotation of carelessness or other negative implications. Likewise, *endpoint* is similar in that in certain settings it has no meaning apart from denoting the limit of something, while in other settings it might have a more coloured meaning. To the contrary, mathematical confusion for the ends of an interval comes from the difference between (and, or $<$ and $<=$. When one of these indicators is used you are including the value at the end of the range. When you use the other indicator, you are specifying that the indicated value is NOT included. If an author says $x<15$, x can never be as large as 15 but must be smaller than 14.99999.... Whereas if $x<=15$, x can be as large as 15.0 (but no larger). This is why the term endpoint is confusing. In statistics, endointsare referred to as "limits" - which implies that the values themselves are included as possible values (which they are). One may loosely define an endpoint as merely a measure of disease-severity. It may be viewed as a standard in the literature. [50] Nevertheless, medically, different diseases have various measures of severity; e.g. for sleep apnea, its measure of severity is the Apnea/hypopnea index (AHI), which is the number of events of apnea/hypopnea per hour. It is a rate, NOT a single point (the endpoint), but is a continuous variable. For another example, in the literature of sleep medicine, AHI is hardly referred as any single point but a rate. [51, 52] Usually, an 'endpoint' or 'end point' is a mark of termination or completion. An 'endpoint' indeed lacks a meaning of the 'measure' or the 'severity' (of diseases). In fact, there are different endpoints in certain diseases, which we need to combine them, and to improve the information content of categorical clinical trial endpoints. [50-52] Hence, the aforementioned discussion has reinforced our consideration that with regard to Crocker et al.'s excellent work [48], it appears to be important to identify a practical proposal about how the crossover data would be analyzed properly in their work that they have reviewed or the data that are belonging to the cases in their Medical Center. The primary analysis of such a study would have to be limited to the randomized patients, as a minimum, in their own data set of the Medical Center. It, as well, appears to be significant in ascertaining that the crossover data would potentially enhance information of estimates with regard to radiological vs. neurosurgical or even medical (specifically, via medications alone), and above, anaesthetic risk respectively or jointly in a variety of combinations. [47]

SECTION 10. ENDOVASCULAR INTERVENTION

At the outset, data analysis of Crocker el al's study revealed that a predominant role for endovascular management for acute rupture (86.6 vs 13.4%) of intracraneal cerebral aneurysm, with an inch by inch greater position for open type microsurgery in the more non-compulsory background (57% endovascular vs 43% surgical). They, in addition, reviewed 66 interventions for arteriovenous malformations (AVM), of which merely 6 were surgical. These information are in contrast against a sample year from 2001 to 2002 (pre-International Subarachnoid Aneurysm Trial), viewing as good as rates of surgically treated aneurysms as related to endovascularly treated aneurysms, nonetheless, an increasing entirely in the number of patients requiring open microneurosurgery. The authors realized that exceptional results for microsurgical clipping compared with endovascular therapy could hence be obtained within the current ambiance. These and previously reported studies profoundly establish a ongoing position for vascular neurosurgery as a subspecialist interest in collaboration with a professional endovascular service and a multidisciplinary squad, which is counting but not limited to neuroradiology and neuroanesthesia. [48]

That being reviewed and then assessed, it would be functional to propose a clinical study where those randomized to the control group could cross over to the interventional group subsequent to some pre-defined period of time or after meeting some sort of reasonable endpoint. With respect to endpoints, there appear to have proper concepts involved. An "endpoint" does not denote the "measure" or "severity" of diseases on it own, at least to this author. There

Neurodiagnostic Pitfalls of CT Scan from Neurosurgical Viewpoint **131**

are certainly different end points in certain diseases, hence we are supposed to combine them and improve the informational content of categorical clinical trial end points. [49] The amount of time and the endpoint would need to be tailored to the particular disease - intracraneal aneurysms or AVM or both, regardless of whether the patients are to be treated in the radiology department or in the Operating Room. At this juncture of discussion, it is worthwhile to notethe clinical exampleexample of Modern Endovascular Techniques.

SECTION 11 A CLINICAL EXAMPLE OF MODERN ENDOVASCULAR TECHNIQUES

That discussed, for another clinical example, it is, as well, worthwhile to note that most recently, Yadia et al. reported their experience with a combined-modality treatment of unruptured carotid-ophthalmic aneurysms over a twelve year period. [55]. Their retrospective review of one-hundred sixty one patients who underwent open, endovascular, or combined treatment of one-hundred seventy aneurysms aneurysms from January 1997 to July 2009 was conducted. They had one-hundred forty-seven aneurysms that were operated through endovascular techniques. Among those one-hundred forty-seven, seventeen aneurysms (10%) were operated with microsurgical clip ligation, as well as six aneurysms (3.5%) were treated with a combined approach of both endovascular techniques and microsurgical clip ligation.

Table 3. Yadia et al's study

Open microsurgical clip ligation	Endovascular	combined treatment
17 aneurysms (10%)	147 aneurysms (86.5%)	6 aneurysms (3.5%)
	81.6% of these 147 aneurysms had evidence of 95% or greater occlusion on initial angiogram	
Major complications rate: 26.1% associated with the initial procedure 6 of 23 (26.1%) open microsurgical procedures including two instances of permanent visual loss.	Major complication rate: 1.4 % associated with the initial procedure. 26 of these aneurysms (18.9%) required further intervention based on early angiographic results.	

132

Bing H. Tang

9 clipped patients had long-term angiographic followup; none required further intervention.		

Among the aneurysms the authors operated on through endovascular techniques alone, 81.6% of aneurysms had proof of 95% or greater stenosis on angiogram. The major complication rate linked with the initial procedure was reported as 1.4%. Major complications took place after 6 of 23 (26.1%) open microsurgical procedures. These complications included two instances of permanent visual loss. Nine clipped patients had long-term angiographic follow-up; none required further intervention. Twenty-six of these aneurysms (18.9%) needed additional intervention based on early angiographic results. [55]

Table 4.Prestigiacomo et alreported 179 consecutive patients with spur-of-the -moment SAH during a period over 36months, as detected by viewing CT and CTA. Patients with negative CTA findings undertook DSA within 24hours of arrangement. All patients who were clinically diagnosed to have angiographically negative SAH undertook follow-up DSA twoweeks later. Among those 179 patients checked by CTA, as the following tabulation

Prestigiacomo et al. reported 179 patients checked by:		
	CTA	MRI
	13 (7%) were negative for aneurysms, arteriovenous malformation or dural fistula on CTA.	The MRI taken in order to exclude thrombosed aneurysms and the repeated angiography at the 2 week interval for follow-up were negative. Those 13 patients were then undertook DSA. There was no new lesions detected on six-vessel-angiography,
	Hence CAT : 1] None false negative rate	
	2] sensitivity 100%, 3] predictive value 100%	

SECTION 11. COMPRESSION OF THE POSTERIOR CRANIAL FOSSA

General speaking, cerebellum lays in the posterior inferior communicaqting artery (PICA) territory distal to the branches to the medulla oblongata. The clinical manifestations commonly consist of rotatory dizziness intensifled by motion, nausea, vomiting, imbalance, and nystagmus. At times, the clinical diagnosis had been a benign labyrinthine disorder, but finally it turned out to be the recognition of a syndrome corresponding to cerebellar infarction in the PICA territory. Hence, it is important that such a diagnosis helps in the differential diagnosis of dizziness. It goes without saying that a situation certainly becomes of crucial importance when cerebellar infarction is the prologue to cerebellar swelling and brain stem compression leading to coma and death unless surgically decompressed. In the past, with the understanding of the definitions for the diagnosis of cerebellar infarction is from the proof of both clinical and laboratory foundation starting from older studies based on the result of autopsy data. In fact, atherosclerotic pathology was usually discovered at bifurcations or even trifurcations and the curvatures of the larger blood vessels. Lehrich et al. reported that since 1960 to 1969 there were four such patients in a 1,000-bed general hospital. [56]. According to the authors, each such patient presented clincially as a posterior fossa mass ompressing brain stem. For the reason that cerebellar infarction may be swiftly fatal without treatment, most physicians are in an attempt to define a syndrome that can be diagnosed early, similar state of affairs hold factual from there even up to state-of-the-art. Because of cerebellar infarction cuts across most attempts to differentiate thrombus from embolus that it as earned its own category, tandem arterial pathology, just as *Tandem Repeat Sequence* in chromosome study, described as a separate entity. [56]

Reviewing mechanisms and locations of cerebral and cerebellar stroke reveals that in order to get a better understanding on what all these cerebral stroke locations mean, the more proximal the location in the blood vessel tree, the more grave the atherosclerotic lesions are. In general, the primary occlusion of arteries, which are distally sited over the cerebral and/or cerebellar cortex are infrequent. The means for getting stroke in atherothrombus likely was at the outset there was perfusion-malfunction at distal portion of the blood vessel. Nonetheless, with some instances, the most important blood vessel occlusion was relatively proximal in the arterial blood vessel tree; some extent of collateral flow was diagnosed between the occlusion and the cerebral area endangered for infarction. However, in the carotid region, these areas were the suprasylvian frontal, central, and parietal parts of the cerebral hemisphere, while in the vertebrobasilar region, the area was the both sided occipital pole. Over and above, vascular occlusion at the location of atherosclerosis, infarcts were, as well, produced by emboli coming form the atheromatous lesions located proximal to if not healthy branches sited more distal in the arterial tree. In this day and age, embolism as of a carotid basis has turned out to be distinguished as another, conceivably more frequent, grounds of stroke in situation of arterial stenosis. [56]

Nowadays, with the help of CTA the early diagnosis will be readily established, hence it can really help for the earlier diagnosis.

SECTION 12. MEDIAL PONTINE STROKE: AN UNUSUAL EXAMPLE

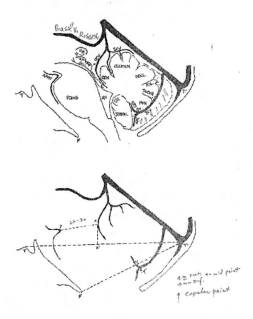

Figure 1. Midline Posterior Fossa View (By Yuen P HuangMD inCerebellopontine Angle Tumors or Acoustic NeuromasLong-Range Management.Morris B. Bender, MD *Arch Otolaryngol.* 1973;97(2):160-165.

The concerns of knowledge of brain-stem anatomy and pathophysiology are ever relevant. This should be important for understanding the very nature of issues such as patients' remaining cognitive and motor abilities subsequent to their brain stem stroke. For instance, Ruhland J, and van Kan PLE reported 'Medial pontine hemorrhagic stroke' in 2003. [57] They recorded an exceptional occasion to scrutinize the motor function of an individual for virtually 6 months subsequent a major bleeding in the medial pontine tegmentum of the brain stem. The aim of their report was to exemplify how acquaintance of brain-stem structure-function relationships, enlightens all of us the neurological examination and diagnostic studies. A right-handed 81–year-old gentleman with high MABP, had a hemorrhagic brain-stem stroke that harshly involves control of posture and the four-limb movements. A quantity of remaining ability to use the right hand and fingers stayed to supply the body trunk, and the right upper limb were stabilized. As far as the range of motion concerned, it had not been weakened. The intellectual capacities were not affected. Memory was intact. The maim fact was due to the sparing of cerebral cortices. Nonetheless, cognitive abilities were obscured by severe destruction in interpersonal contact as a consequence of widespread injury to cranial nerve structures. CT scans helped to identified that the hematoma crossed the midline and was restricted to the area of medial pontine tegmentum.

Neurodiagnostically speaking, in the authors' report, such an excellent CT scan finding has done a great job without leaving any neurodiagnostic pitfalls. [57]

SECTION 13. MIDBRAIN STROKE ARISING FROM BOTH THALAMI

Recently, Muhammad Khalil, Tayyaba Gul Malik and Khalid Farooq and the Editors of JCPSP published their case report, which shows multiple infarcts affecting both thalami and extending caudally into midbrain. Their case presents a diverse clinical manifestation following another quite different type of midbrain stroke. [58]

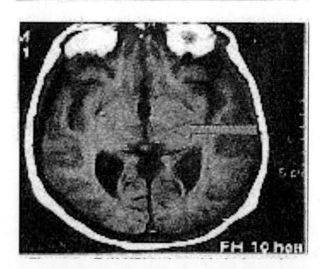

Figure 2. MRI brain (axial view) showing hypointense areas close to midline at the level of thalamomesencephalic junction.

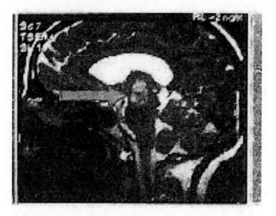

Figure 3. MRI brain (sagital view) showing infarcts in thalamus and midbrain.

SECTION 14. VESTIBULAR SCHWANNOMA

Acoustic neuromas, also known as vestibular schwannomas, are non-malignant tumors of the 8th cranial nerve. Commonly they arise from the covering cells (Schwann cells) of the inferior vestibular nerve [59 Komatsuzaki and Tsunoda, 2001], [60 Krais, 2007). They may, as well, arise within the labyrinth [61 Neff et al, 2003].

As nowadays, CT and MRI scans become more commonly used, there is more acoustics neuroma being discovered accidentally and unintentionally. For incidence, a person who has a migraine headache, the physician might get an MRI scan, which reveals an acoustic neuroma. Or someone who suffered from an automobile accident, might get an MRI scan, which reveals an acoustic neuroma.

Nonetheless, there are still some other neurodiagnostic pitfalls involved. In fact, CT scans enhenced with intravenous injection of contrastrast material are poor diagnosisic tests for diagnosing acoustic neuromas, as CT scans have a high false negative rate (37%). [62 Shneider et al] In persons with metal in vital places -- such as a pacemaker, sometimes CT scan is the only test available, though there are definitely neurodiagnostic pitfalls involved.

Molecular Biology of NF2

Pertaining to molecular biology, conscientious to genotype-phenotype correlation in NF2, It is understood that the splice-site mutations [63 Huttons] associated with various phenotypes, which vary from severe to nonsymptomatic. As well as interfamily dissimilarity, phenotypic disparities are scrutinized within families. Mutations downstream from exon 8 (as contrast to intron, extron is a segment of a gene, which is decoded to provide a messenger RNA or mature RNA product) result more frequently in meek phenotypes of NF2. This designates that splice-site modification is a comparatively ordinary cause of NF2 and that splice-site modification does not give the impression of any other mutations: the clinical outcomes of splice-site mutations in the NF2 gene are fairly changeable. For this very reason, the enormously mounting volume of information on genotype/phenotype association in NF2 has been distended and lengthened. [63, 64 (Tang 2004)]

Section 15. An Example of Uncommon Extracranial Tumor

For example, Tsai, Lin and Tseng in 2008 reported a case of Hemangiopericytoma in the Right Buccal Area. [65]

It has been noted that Hemangiopericytomas (HPCs) are uncommon tumor of blood vessel origin that take place in the cranial and cervical regions. These tumors result from capillary pericytes and are easier said than done to differentiate from other tumors of blood vessel origin. Description is reliant on histological examination. The uncommon happening of these neoplasms and their changeable malignant and latent potential has restricted to the efforts trying to typify their clinical role and behavior. Lin et al. in 2008 reported a case of HPC located in the right buccal area of a young woman. Treatment included radical tumor excision and reconstruction using a free myocutaneous flap. At four-year post-operative follow-up, there was no evidence of recurrence, though noticeably, there are high incidence of local recurrence. CT scan evidence, which reveals that the mass lesion is protruding from the middle craneal fossa to the submandibular region of the right buccal membrtane.

Without any neurodiagnostic pitfalls, CT scan report of this case reveals as following:

There was a giant and well-enhanced mass lesion about 5.5 x 4.8 cm in size in the right buccal space with superior extension to the right middle craneal, namely, infratemporal fossa, medial to the masticator space and retromolar region, and inferior to the lower gum region. There were associated with prominent vascular enhancement surrounding this mass lesion and containing with cystic part.

Pathological Description

Microscopically, it shows oval or spindle tumor cells with plenty eosionphilic cytoplasm arranged in multinodular pattern with so-called *staghorn vessels*. The mitoses is scanty. Focal vascular permeation is noted. The overlying squamous epithelium is intact.

Immunohistochemical study

Immunohistochemical study shows vimentin(+), cytokeration(-), EMA(-), S-100(-), smooth muscle actin(-), desmin(-), CD34(-). The picture is in favor of hemangiopericytoma. [65]

Vimentin is a type III intermediate filament protein that is expressed in mesenchymal cells. Any tumor cells (or normal cells) with mesenchymal differentiation can express vimentin, including the case just reported here, hemangiopericytoma (HPC), which is now believed to originate from pericytes surrounding the blood vessel. of HPC is considered. Other possible tumors with vimentin expression include: solitary fibrous tumor, and glomangioma.[66]

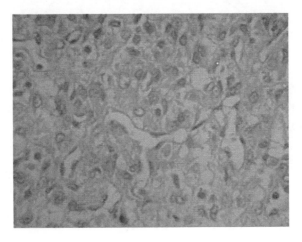

Figure 4. Tsai' et al's study on HPC.

Section 16. A Neurodiagnostic Pitfall of CT Scan, Assessed from Neurosurgical View Point, Specific in Children's Spine : Children's Sciwora Syndrome: (Spinal Cord Injury without Radiologic Abnormality)

Each year, more than 20,000 children expire as a result of injuries attributable to motor vehicle accidents, falls and bicycles [66 Stein SC 1]. Head injury is, thus far, cause of morbidity and mortality in children between 1 and 14 years, and amounts up to 70% of all children's injury deaths (2).

In cerebral contusion, or even anemia or in its most serious form, disseminated intravascular coagulation (DIC) [1 – 6] exposures subendothelial collagen and releases tissue. Thromboplastin [1, 2], hence leads to hemorrhage and thrombosis. Whether coagulopathy takes place as a biological and clinical marker of severe head injury and brain trauma [67 Tang JAMC], or, in fact, contributes to secondary brain injury is less important to be debated in viewing with the following fact specific in children's traumatic spinal condition, which deserve our special consideration indeed. [68]

It is very important to be aware of Children's Sciwora syndrome' which has been reported by what has been showed in the following table merely for the aim of easy glancing:

Table 5. SciworaSyndrome

15 Children	Parethesis	Lehermitte'sign	Recurrence	CT/CTA scan
15 children have delayed onset of delayed onset of neurological deficits	9 of these have paresthesia	subjective paresis and Lhermitte's sign 30 mins to 4 days prior to neurological deterioration.	of these children have recurrent Sciwora 3 to 10 days after the original SCIWORA	Spine condition of these children is incipiently unstable.

Though the spine condition of these children is incipiently unstable in the clinical manifestation, nonetheless, the neurodiagnostic pitfalls of CT scans include but not limiting to the aforementioned neuroradiological finding indeed warrants our serious attention.

SECTION 17. CONCLUSION

Now we are living in this society where we have already gained a lot of benefits by using CT scans; nonetheless, we are, as well, encountering some neurodiagnostical pitfalls arising from using it, just as having been outlined and discussed respectively as aforementioned as per this author's personal perspective, from a neurosurgical viewpoint.

Various sections have been presented in this chapter. They are expected by this author to be informative and helpful to all sereaders.

ACKNOWLEDGMENT

The author is grateful to Vice President of University, Dr. Wu Trongneng, as well, to Dr. Tsai Ming-Hsui, Professor and Chairman, Department of Otolaryngology, China Medical University Hospital, Taiwan, and his coauthors for allowing this author to use their intereting figues of an article entitled "Hemagiopericytoma in the Right Buccal Area". Likewise, thanks go to Drs. Muhammad Khalil, Tayyaba Gul Malik and Khalid Farooq, as well, Editors of JCPSP for their permission to use the figures of an article entitled "Weber's Syndrome with Vertical Gaze Palsy".

This author, as well, thank all the Editors and authors of various journals for their respective and informative articles, which all have all together made this review available today.

For the critical reading, this author thanks his dear eldest son, Mr. Jack Tang, B.S.

For the editorial assistance for the preparation of this chapter, this author is grateful to his dear niece Miss Carolyn Uy, B. S. in Manila.

REFERENCES

1. Tang B., McKenna P., Rovit R. Primary Fibrinolytic Syndrome Associated with Subarachnoid Hemorrhage. Angiology, Nov. 1973, 627-34

2. Tang B. Recent Advances in Neurotraumatology Edited by.Chiu, Wen-Da. Nov. 20, 1999, MonduzziEditore, Italy.137—143 , seven pages.

3. Moltke, P.: Plasminogen Activator in Leptomeninges, Proc. Soc. Exp. Biol. Med. 98:377, 1958.

4. Tang, B. Disseminated Intravascular Coagulation and the Neurosurgeon In Chiu WD (ed) International Conference in Recent Advances in Neurotraumatology. Bologna, Italy. 137- 8

5. Sherry, S. Fibrinolysis, Annual Review of Medicine, Vol.19: 247, Edited by Graff, A.C. and Creger, W.P., Palo Alto. Annual Reviews Inc., 1968.

6. Ratnoff, D.D.: Some relationships among hemostasis, fibrinolyticphenomence, immunity and the inflammatory process. Advances Immun. 10: 145, 1969.

7. Abildgaard, C.F.: Recognition and treatment of intravascular coagulation, J. Pediat., 74:163,1969.

8. Harsaway, R.M.: Syndromes of Disseminated Intravascular Coagulation, Springfield, I11., Charles C Thomas, 1966.

9. Ingram, G.I.C.: The defibrination syndrome, in Recent Advances in Blood Coagulation, edited by Poller, L. London, Chruchill, p.263, 1969.

10. McGehie, W.G., Rapaport, s.d. and Hjort, P.: Intravascular coagulation in fulminant meningocoiemia, Ann. Int. Med., 67:250, 1967.

11. McKay, D.G.: Disseminated Intravascular Coagulation. An Intermediary Mechanism of Disease. New York, Hoeber, 1965.

12. Merskey, G., Johnson, A.J., Kleiner, G.J. and Wohl, H.: The defibrination syndrome: clinical features and laboratory diagnosis. Brit. J. Haemat. 13: 528.

13. Rodriguez-Erdmann, F.: bleeding due to increased intravascular blood coagulation: hemorrhagic syndromes caused by consumption of blood clotting factors (consumption coagulopathies). New Eng. J. of Med. 273: 1370, 1965.

14. Rosner, F. And Ritz, N.D.: The defrination syndrome, Archives of Internal Medicine, 117: 17, 1966.

15. Verstraete, M., Vermylen, C., Cermylen, J. and Vandenbroucke, J.: Excessive consumption of blood coagulation components as cause of hemorrhagic diathesis, Amer. J. Med., 38: 899, 1965.

16. Schneck, S.A. and Von Kaulla K.N.: Fibronolysis and the nervous system, Neurology 11:959, 1962.

17. Von Kaulla K.N.: Fibronolysis and the nervous system, Neurology 11:959, 1962.

18 Heilbrum, M.P.: Regional cerebral blood flow in subarachnoid hemorrhage, J. Neurosurg., 37:38, 1972.

Neurodiagnostic Pitfalls of CT Scan from Neurosurgical Viewpoint   143

19. Petruk, K.C., West, G.R., McIntyre, J.W., Overton, T.R., Bryce, K.A.W.: Cerebral blood flow following induces subarachnid hemorrhage in monkeys, J Neurosurg., 37: 316-324, 1972.

20. Kivan, H.C., and McFadzcan, A.J.S.: Plasma fibrinolytic activity induced by ischaemia, Clin. Sci., 15:245, 956.

21. Miner ME, Kaufman HH, Graham SH, Haar FH, Goldenberg PL. Intravascular fibrinolytic syndrome following head injury in childrens' frequency and prognostic implications. J. Pediatr 1982; 100: 687-691.

22. PONDAAG. DISSEMINATED INTRAVASCULAR COAGULATION RELATED TO OUTCOME IN HEAD INHURY. ACTA NEUROCHIR SUPPL (WIEN) 1978; 28: 98-102

23. Greenberg, J. Cohen WA, Cooper PR. The "hyperacute" extraaxial intracranial hematoma: computed tomographic findings and clinical significance. Neurosurgery 1985; 17: 46-56

24. Boyko OB, Cooper DF, Grossman CB. Contrast-enhanced CT of acute isodense subdural hematoma. AJNR 1991; 12: 341-343

25. Boroojerdi, B, Toshikatsu Yamamoto, GnterSchumpe, Thomas Schockert. Treatment Of Stroke-Related Motor Impairment By Yamamoto New Scalp Acupuncture (YNSA): An Open, Prospective, Topometrically Controlled Study. Medical Accupuncture. 17;1

26. Php de Aguiar, Paulo Henrique Pires, Zicarelli, Carlos Alexandre Martins; Aires, Rogério, Santiago, Natally Marques, Tahara, Adriana; Simm, RenataIsolan, Gustavo Rassier. Posterior Communicating Artery Aneurysms: Technical Pitfalls. Neurosurgery Quarterly: June 2010 - 20;2:74-81

27. Hunt WE, Hess RM. "Surgical risk as related to time of intervention in the repair of intracranial aneurysms. Journal of Neurosurgery 1968 Jan;28(1):14-20.

28. Hunt WE, Meagher JN, Hess RM. "Intracranial aneurysm. A nine-year study. Ohio State Medical Journal 1966 Nov;62(11):1168-71.

29. Ng Shu-Hang, Ho-Fai Wongb, Sheung-Fat Kob, Chi-Ming Leeb, Pao-Sheng Yenb, Yau-YauWaib and Yung-Liang Wang. CT angiography of intracranial aneurysms: advantages and pitfalls. 1997.

30. Bash S, Villablanca JP, Jahan R. Intracranial vascular stenosis and occlusive disease: Evaluation with CT angiography, MR angiography, and digital subtraction angiography. *AJNR Am J Neuroradiol. * 2005;26:1012-1021.

31. Nguyen-Huynh MN, Wintermark M, English J, et al. How accurate is CT angiography in evaluating intracranial atherosclerotic disease? Stroke.2008; 39:1184-1188.

32. Anderson, Glenn B. ; Findlay, J. Max ; Steinke, David E. ; Ashforth Robert. Experience with Computed Tomographic Angiography for the Detection of Intracranial Aneurysms in the Setting of Acute Subarachnoid Hemorrhage. Neurosurgery September 1997 - Volume 41 - Issue 3 - pp 522-528

33. Howington J., Scott C. Kutz, Gregory E. Wilding, Deepak Awasthi Cocaine use as a predictor of outcome in aneurismal subarachnoid hemorrhage J Neurosurg 99:271–275, 2003.

34 Lange RA, Cigarroa RG, Yancy CW Jr, Willard JE, Popma JJ, Sills MN, McBride W, Kim AS, Hillis LD : Cocaine-induced coronary-artery vasoconstriction. N Engl J Med.1989 Dec 7;321(23):1557-62

35 Fisher CM, Kistler JP, Davis JM: Relation of cerebral vasospasm to subarachnoid hemorrhage visualized by computerized tomographic scanning. Neurosurgery 6:1-9, 1980 Pubmed

36. TetsuyoshiHoriuchi. Anteriororsubtemporal approach for the posterior communicating artery aneurysm protruding posteriorly. Neurosurgical Review Volume 30, Number 3, 203-207, DOI: 10.1007/s10143-007-0083-7

37. Oyesiku NM, Colohan AR, Barrow DL: Cocaine-induced aneurysmal rupture: an emergent negative factor in the natural history of intracranial aneurysms? Neurosurgery 32:518-526, 1993 Pubmed

38. Salom JB, Torregrosa G, Barbera MD: Effects of cocaine on human and goat isolated cerebral arteries. Drug Alcohol Depend 42:65-71, 1996 Pubmed

39. Simpson RK Jr, Fischer DK, Narayan RK: Intravenous cocaine abuse and subarachnoid haemorrhage: effect on outcome. Br J Neurosurg 4:27-30, 1990 Pubmed

40. Weiss RD, Gawin FH: Protracted elimination of cocaine metabolites in long-term high-dose cocaine abusers. Am J Med 85:879-880, 1988 Pubmed

41. Caplan LR, Hier DB, Banks G: Current concepts of cerebrovascular disease--stroke: stroke and drug abuse. Stroke 13:869-872, 1982 Pubmed

42. Levine SR, Brust JC, Futrell N: A comparative study of the cerebrovascular complications of cocaine: alkaloidal versus hydrochloride--a review. Neurology 41:1173-1177, 1991

43 Tang B: Cocaine use as the Predicator of Subarachnoid Hemorrage . J. of Neurosurgery, Vol.102, p 961-2, May, 2005
***SCI

44. Trial on endovascular treatment of unruptured intracranial aneurysms (TEAM)
http://www.sfnv-france.com/pdf/etude-clinique-team.pdf accessed on 30 April 2011.

45.Altman DG. Practical statistics for medical research Chapman & Hall, London and Newe York, 611 pages
1991.

46. Senn, S: Cross-over trials in clinical research - (Statistics in Practice) 2002, 2nd ed. Chichester: John Wiley & Sons, Ltd.

47. Crocker M, Corns R, Hampton T, Deasy N, Tolias CM. Vascular neurosurgery following the International Subarachnoid Aneurysm Trial: modern practice reflected by subspecialization. J Neurosurg. 2008 Dec;109(6):992-7

48. Crocker M, Corns R, Hampton T, Deasy N, Tolias CM. Vcular neurosurgery following the International Subarachnoid Aneurysm Trial: modern practice reflected by subspecialization. J Neurosurg. 2008 Dec; 109(6):992-7   crocker

49. ang, B. Crossover trials, J. of Neurosurgery August 2009 Volume 111, Number 2 (doi: 10.3171/jns.2005.102.5.0961)

50 Tang, B. Biostatistics with Neurosurgical Importance. J Neurosurg. 168; 1256-1261, June, 2008 SCI

51.Tang B. Living on a biological clock: age-related functional changes of sleep homeostat in 65 to 88.5 year old people. Sleep and Biological Rhythms 2007; 5: 180-95 (Blackwell publication)

52. Tang B. Letter to Editor. JAMC. 2008;20;2

53. Heros RC: Case volume and mortality. J Neurosurg 99:805– 806, 2003

54. Heros RC: Clip ligation or coil occlusion?. J Neurosurg 104:341–343, 2006

55. Yadla S, Campbell P, BartoszGrobenly B, Jallo J, Gonzalez L, Rosenwasser R, Jabbour R. Open and endovascular treatment of unruptured carotid ophthalmic aneurysms: Clinical and radiographic outcome. Neurosurgery .2011.jan 26 (Epub ahead of print) .

56. Lehrich J, Winkler G, Ojemann R: Cerebellar infarction with brainstem compression. J Neurosurg 17:7

57.Ruhland J, and van Kan PLE reported 'Medial pontine hemorrhagic stroke' in 2003.

58. Muhammad Khalil, TayyabaGul Malik and Khalid Farooq. Weber's Syndrome with Vertical Gaze Palsy" by Muhammad Khalil, TayyabaGul Malik and Khalid Farooq published in JCPSP 2009 Vol:19(10) 668-669

59. Komatsuzaki A, Tsunoda A. Nerve origin of the acoustic neuroma. J LaryngolOtol 2001 May;115(5):376-9

60. Khrais T, Romano G, SannaMJ . Nerve origin of vestibular schwannoma: a prospective study..Laryngol Otol. 2007 Nov 27;

61. Neff, Brian A; Welling, D Bradley; Akhmametyeva, Elena; Chang, Long-Sheng. Tumors of The Ear & Cranial Base. The Molecular Biology of Vestibular Schwannomas: Dissecting the Pathogenic Process at the Molecular Level. Otology &Neurotology: 2006 - 27;2, 97-208

62. Shneider B, Schneider AB, Ron E, Lubin J. Acoustic neuromas following childhood radiation treatment for benign conditions of the head and neck. NeuroOncol. 2007 Dec 13

63. Yohay K. Neurofibromatosis types 1 and 2. Neurologist. 2006 Mar;12(2):86-93.

64. Tang B. Predictors of Vestibular Schwannoma Growth in patients with Neurofibromatosis Type 2   J. of Neurosurgey Volume 100 , p. 734, April, 2004   SCI == 2.286

65. Lin C, Tseng, Tsai Ming-Hsui. Hemagiopericytoma in the Right Buccal Area. Mid-Taiwan J. of Medicine Sep 2008;13:156-60

66. Catalano PJ, Brandwein M, Shah DK, Urken ML, Lawson W, Biller HF.   Sinonasalhemangiopericytomas: a   clinicopathologic   and immunohistochemical study of seven cases.   Head Neck. 1996 Jan-Feb;18(1):42-53.

67.WWW.consumerfed.org/elements/www.consumerfed.org/file/health/Final_ATVReportLinks.pdf (accessed October 25, 2011)

68 Tang, B. The critical analysis on diagnosis of Dissinated Intravascular Coagulation with Screening Tests-a Scoring System and Related Literature Review.JAMC Oct-Dec 2007; 19(4):112-120

69   Pang D, Pollack IF. Spinal cord injury without radiographic abnormality in children--the SCIWORA syndrome. J Trauma. 1989 May;29(5):654-64

In: CT Scans
Editors: V. E. Perkel et al.

ISBN 978-1-62100-319-9
©2012 Nova Science Publishers, Inc.

Chapter 4

NEURODIAGNOSTIC PITFALLS OF CT SCANS FROM NEURORADIOLOGICAL VIEWPOINT: *A PERSONAL PERSPECTIVE*

Bing H Tang[a, b] and Eve Tiu[a]

[a]Reseach & Ethics, Danville, Calif., U. S.
[b]Institute of Biological Chemistry, Academia Sinica, Taiwan

ABSTRACT

CT scanning, also being called as CAT scanning, is a noninvasive medical test that helps physicians diagnose and treat medical conditions. It combines special x-ray equipment with sophisticated computers to produce multiple images or pictures of the inside of the body. These cross-sectional images of the area being studied can then be examined on a computer monitor, printed or transferred to a CD. CT scans of internal organs, bones, soft tissue and blood vessels provide greater clarity and reveal more details than regular x-ray exams. Radiologists can more easily diagnose problems such as cancers, cardiovascular disease, infectious disease, appendicitis, trauma and musculoskeletal disorders. It is invaluable in diagnosing and treating brain and spinal problems and injuries to the hands, feet and other skeletal structures because it can clearly show even very small bones as well as surrounding tissues such as muscle and blood vessels. As to the CT scan diagnosis of blood vessel diseases, it is very complex for Central Nervous System. There are diagnostic pitfalls of CT scans in this System. Hence, such a discussion posted in this article will be carried out from Neuroradiological viewpoint.

Methods

1. Reappraisal of Primary Fibrinolytic Syndromes associoated with subarachnoid Hemorrage, which has been the first report in medical literature since 1973.
2. Some review and analysis of Isodensity in CT scans with Bilateral Cerebral Subdural Hematomas (SDH).
3. Some review and analysis of Cerebral Posterior Circulation Vasculature
4. Some review and analysis of CTA, MRA, TOF-MRA, DAS, and MDTC.

Result

Primary Fibrinolytic Syndrome Assocoiated with Subarachniod Hemorrage (SDH) that this author, with two coauthors, reported in 1973 appears to be the initial report on this syndrome in medical literature. As well, the midbrain and thalamic infarcts associated with subarachnoid hemorrhage reported in the identical case were arising from the rupture of a posterior communicating artery aneurysm. (1)

Cerebral Vertebrobasilar Circulation was involved in that case. The so-called 'polar artery' is a synonym of the posterior communicating artery, in which the location of this artery is the similar site of the rupture of an aneurysm reported elsewhere by this author. [2-5].

As a contrast to what happened in the early 1970s, nowadays we are living in a society where we are not only gaining a lot of benefits, but also encountering some neurodiagnostical pitfalls arising from using CT scans.

Review and evaluation of CT scan's neurodiagnostic pitfalls are provided in this chapter.

Keywords: Arterial Venous malformation (AVM) posterior inferior cerebellar artery, Computed tomography (CT), Computed tomographic angiography (CTA), RF (Radiofrequency, Time-of-flight magnetic resonance angiography (TOF-MRA)

ABBREVIATIONS

ASIR Adaptive statistical iterative reconstruction
AVM Arterial Venous malformation
CD Compact Disc
CE Cerebral Edema
CSF Cerebral Spinal Fluid
CT Computerized Tomography
DIC Disseminated Coagulation
EDH Epidural Hematoma
FBP Filtered-back Projection
FDP Fibrin Degradation Products
GCS Glasgow Coma Score
GOS Glasgow Outcome Scale
HCT Hematocrit
PLT Platelet
PT Prothrombin Time
PTT Partial Thromboplastin Time
ICH Intracranial Hemorrhage
IVH Intraventricular Hemorrhage
MABP Mean arterial blood pressure
MDCT Multidetector
NPS Noise Power Spectrum
SAH Subarachnoid Hemorrhage
SDH Subdural Hematoma
Tissue plasminogen activator (tPA)
TOF Time of flight

INTRODUCTION

CT scanning, also being called as CAT scanning, is a noninvasive medical test that helps physicians diagnose and treat medical conditions. It combines special radiological equipment with sophisticated computers to produce multiple images or pictures of the inside of body. These cross-sectional images of the area being studied can then be examined on a computer monitor, printed or transferred to a CD. CT scans of internal organs, bones, soft tissue and blood vessels provide greater clarity and reveal more details than regular x-ray examination. Radiologists can more easily diagnose problems such as cancers, cardiovascular disease, infectious disease, appendicitis, trauma and musculoskeletal disorders. It is invaluable in diagnosing and treating spinal problems and injuries to the hands, feet and other skeletal structures because it can clearly show even very small bones as well as surrounding tissues such as muscle and blood vessels. As to the CT scan diagnosis of blood vessel diseases, it is very complex for Central Nervous System. There are diagnostic pitfalls of CT scans in this System. Hence, such a discussion focused on this chapter will be starting from two examplified fibrinolytic cases, then The Post-CT-Scanner Era, and carrying out from Neuroradiological viewpoint, followed with the discussion on computed tomography angiography (CTA), TOF MRA with its relationship to Neurosurgical Planning, CTA for diagnosis of carotid artery stenosis/occlusion, and MR angiography. Comparison of positive predictive values between CTA and MRA in some exmaplifid study is to be addressed. Signal loss in TOF MRA is to be discussed as well. Drawbacks and mistakes of CTA are to be outlined. An introduction of 179 consecutive patients with spur-of-the-moment subarachnoid hemorrhage (SAH) during a period over 36 months is provided; the SAH was detected by viewing CT and CTA, given those patients with negative CTA findings undertook digital subtraction angigraphy (DSA) within 24 hours.

In the final Section, there will be a briefing of the cutting edge 'Three dimensional noise power spectrum applied on clinical MDCT scanners: effects of reconstruction algorithms and reconstruction filters'. Noticeably, MDCT is the abbreviation of Multidetector.

SECTION 1

Two Exemplified Cases of Fibrinolytic Syndrome

1. Primary Fibrinolytic Syndrome Associated with Subarachnoid Hemorrhage

First Admission

A 62-year-old Caucasian woman, was admitted to a Medical Center of New York City on July 12,1972, with a one-month history of headache, stiffness and pain in the neck, bilateral buttock and right leg pain, difficulty in walking and double vision.

The MABP was 154/90 mmHg. There were no other outstanding physical or neurological findings. Lumbar puncture was carried out, which revealed cerebrospinal fluid pressures (CSF) were normal initially, the repeated specimen of CSF fluid was xanthochromic with protein of 80 mg%. The following CSF fluid was clear.

Second Admission of the Same Patient

On September 13, 1972, the patient was brought to Hospital in a lethargic state, having been found lying on the floor of her apartment for an undetermined length of time. She was confused, disoriented, dehydrated, and only able to respond to simple commands. Blood pressure was 130/90 mm Hg. Positive physical findings were several small areas of ecchymosis over the right leg, and a third degree burn, sized 5x3 cams over the right lateral thigh. Neurological examination revealed bilateral papilledema with a peripapillary fundal hemorrhage on the right, nuchal rigidity, right hemiparesis, and a dilated right pupil were noted. Both pupils reacted to light.

Laboratory findings revealed decreased platelets (PLT), anisocytosis and ecchinocytosis of red blood cells as well as a shift to the left and toxic granulation of the neutrophils were noted on the peripheral blood smear. Urea nitrogen was 180mg%, and sodium 121 meq/L. Cerebrospinal fluid (CSF) pressure was 220 mm. The fluid appeared xanthochromic with protein of 180 mg%, red blood count of 1000 per mm^3 and no white blood cells found.

The initial studies of hemostatic function included as following: activated partial thromboplastin time (PPT) 36 seconds – control 35 seconds); PT prothrombin time (21 seconds—control 11 seconds); thrombin time (30 seconds—control 20 seconds); stypven time (21 seconds—control 20 seconds); euglobulin lysis time (35 minutes—control more than 90 minutes); fibrin plate lysis (118 mm²--control 50mm²); fibrinogen degradation products (FDP) 60ug/ml—control 16 ug/ml.) and fibrinogen (90mg%--normal 150-350 mg%).

The left carotid and right vertebral angiograms via catheter revealed multiple areas of narrowing of cerebral vessels secondary to spasm. The narrowing of the cerebral vessels was most prominent over the proximal portions of anterior and middle cerebral arteries of the left side. Severe CE, TCH, IVH, and spasm of the left vertebral artery were noted and this vessel was only filled by the right subclavian route. A small aneurysm was seen in the region of the left posterior communicating artery.

One hour later, after the patient being returned to the ward, the patient was found to be flaccid, unresponsive, diaphoretic and ashen. Her blood pressure at this time, MABP was 70/40 mm Hg and pulse rate was70 per minute. Generalized ccchymosis of the skin was present and there was marked swelling and ecchymosis over the left femoral region at the site of the retrograde femoral catheterization. The patient was treated with steroids, blood transfusion, plasma, epsilon aminocaproic acid and vitamin K1, but remained comatose and expired twenty-four hours after that second admission.

Post-Mortem Examination

At post-mortem examination, the significant gross findings included: (a) a small ruptured aneurysm of the left posterior communicating artery, left posterior communicating artery with extensive hemorrhage into the subarachnoid space (SAH). The lumen of the residual aneurismal sac was filled with firmly adherent clotted blood (b) diffuse swelling of the left cerebral hemisphere (CE); (c) a hematoma extending from the region of the left femoral artery to the abdominal wall and retropubic space; (d) three hundred ml. of unclotted blood in the peritoneal cavity; and (e) extensive hemorrhage and exxhymosis of the skin, mucous membranes, pericardium, perirenal and perigastric tissue.

Microscopic Finding

Notable microscopic findings were: (a) an aneurysm of the left posterior communicating artery with residual thrombus. The thrombus showed advanced organization at the periphery but no organization centrally; (b) cellular bone marrow with normal erythroid and myeloid tissue but absent megakaryocytes; and no evidence of peripheral vascular thrombi nor arteriolar fibrin deposition. Neither the renal arterioles nor the glomeruli showed any fibrin deposition.

Two categories of tissue activators have also been identified an activator present in endothelial cells of blood vessels, and an activator present in the lysosomal granules of cells obtained from a variety of tissue. Of particular significance in this case is the fact that large quantities of plasminogen activator are present in the leptomeninges of brain. [1]

Fibronolytic disorders may result from either primary activation of the fibrinolytic system [1] or by secondary activation of this system as a consequence of intravascular coagulation [2].

Interim Discussion

This patient had at least two episodes of SAH from a ruptured aneurysm of the left posterior communicating artery over a two month period. The second episode of SAH was complicated by defective hemostasis due to increased systemic fibrinolysis. Despite the theoretical possibility of increased systemic fibrinolytic activity associated with SAH bleeding, there are no previous reports of such an occurrence in the literature.

In retrospect, there seemed to be two separate events that influenced the increased fibrinolytic activity in this patient. The initial event was most likely connected in some way with the rupture of an aneurysm and subsequent subarachnoid hemorrhage. The second event was related to the performance of the cerebral angiogram catheterization.

Fibrinolysis in man is an important homeostatic process [3, 4] and serves primarily to limit fibrin deposition. Fibrinolysis is mediated by plasmin. Two categories of tissue activators have also been identified; an activator present in endothelial cells of blood vessels, and another activator present in the lysosomal granules of cells obtained from a variety of tissue (tPA). Of particular significance in this case is the observation of large quantities of plasminogen activator (tPA) is present in leptomeninges of the brain.

Secondary fibrinolytic disorders are found in association with disseminated intravascular coagulation (DIC), an intermediate phase of a wide variety of diseases. DIC appears to be, as well, degeneration of thrombin activities arising from plasminogen. It is possible that either the inflammatory reaction caused by blood in the subarachnoid space or ischemia, caused by SAH, might have initiated the release of plasminogen activators from the leptomeninges and stimulated plasmin formation. [1, 5]

The relationship between contrast radiographic studies and systemic fibrinolysis is not entirely clear, but these diagnostic manipulations may at times be associated with transient ischemia of the cerebral circulation. Cerebral ischemia in turn has been noted to cause the release of tPA. [1]

2. A 74-Year-Old Male of Subarachnoid Hemorrage

The patient, a 74 years old Taiwanese male fell down from the motor vehicle accident on 6, 11, 1998, complained of headache, dizziness and left sided weakness. CT scan was done on August 11, 1998 at a regional teaching hospital in Mid-Taiwan. It revealed a right sided subdural hematoma (SDH),

Glascow Coma Scale (GCS) (GOS) showed: E4V5M4 = 13. On August 14, 1998 the patient was operated on, the right parietal chronic and subacute SDH 150 ml with subdural membrane were removed. Post-operatively, the patient was doing very well, he even removed endotracheeal tube, nasogastric (NG) tube and arterial line by himself. His left hemiparesis improved.

On August, 22, 1998, post-operative 7th day, the patient vomited three times; he was lethargic but could be wakeed; his GCS was E3V3M3. His left hemiparesis got worse. Left Basbinski sign was positive. Right arm had ecchymosis 23 by 5 cm.

On the same day, the liquid collected out of the suction of NG tube showed occult blood. Cerebral CT scan revealed no IVH and no ICH either but right frontotemporal acute SDH, which was removed in the amount of 15 ml. There was no EDH. At that juncture, the CT scan finding appeared to be uneventful, which was straightforward without any pitfalls.

Laboratory Finding at That Juncture Revealed as Following

His HCT was steadily decreased.

Prothrombin time (PT) 16.6 (normal range 12-16), and partial thrombin time (PTT) 31.6 (24-40), both test results were within normal ranges.

PLT counts were carried out on August 22, 1998, which showed a decreasing from 120,000 to 103,000 mm^3; on the following day, it further dropped to 103, 000 mm^3, and finally decreased to 101,000 mm^3. C-Reactive Protein test revealed 8.2 8 mg/dl on August 13, 1998 (The normal value should be less than 0.8 u mg/dl.)

Also due to ecchymotic areas were over bilateral arms and legs, right forearm (with petechiae), chest, and back, the clinical impression of DIC was established, the patient was then transferred to a Mid-Taiwan medical center for further hematological management. [2]

SECTION 2

The Post CT Scanner Era

The introduction of CT scanners, as well, its supplementing the traditional catheter angiography helps for refined image of the 3-dimensional anatomy. It can, as well, supply surgical information about the neck, calcification and

Neurodiagnostic Pitfalls of CT Scans ...

thrombosed portion of an aneurysm and its relationship to the surrounding anatomical structure.

With escalating degree of improvement in CT scanners, it has increased the extent of greater craniocaudal exposure at increasingly quicker scanning time and much better resolution. For stroke patients the contemporary high-tech CTA imaging relies on 64-slice CT scanner, which can scan blood vessels in about an order of 3 to 4 sec at submillimeter isotropic resolution.

Therefore, the acquisition time is considerably shorter than single-slice CTA and 4-slice CTA respectively. This, as well, imply that less contrast material is needed, and it is meaning that on the 64-slice CTA, the circulating time within the blood vessel is less than that of single- or 4-slice CTA. The arterial pseudo-occlusion, a type of flow artifact sustained by fast CT scanning is to be discussed.

Noted that ever since December of 1997, Ng et al. reported that in order to decide the efficacy of clinical application of computed tomography angiography (CTA) in the evaluation of cerebral aneurysms, they analyzed the outcome of 26 patients with 30 surgical proven intracranial aneurysms underwent both CT angiography and catheter cerebral angiography, from the period starting October 1994 through April 1996. After those two methods were reviewed independently, and then compared with each other, they discovered that comparing with catheter angiography, CT angiography was much better than catheter angiograph with regard to demonstrating the aneurysmal neck in seven aneurysms. There was merely one case appeared to be inferior to catheter angiograph. On CT angiograms, the thrombosed part, as well as, the calcification portion of aneurysms was obviously illustrated. Hence, CT angiography, as well, assisted in distinguishing doubly knitted vascular loops from aneurysms.

In their CTA study, Ng et al. discovered that one posterior communicating arterial aneurysm was missed and another anterior choroidal artery aneurysm was misdiagnosed as a posterior communicating artery aneurysm. In this context, it is noticeable that there were two patients in whom the infundibulum of an orbitofrontal artery was misdiagnosed as an anterior communicating artery aneurysm. [6]

It thus appears to be reasonable for the authors to conclude that CTA has the advantage for at least:

1) CT can complement conventional catheter angiography with its clearer illustration of the 3-dimensional anatomy.

2) CT can provide surgical information about the aneurysmal neck *per se*.

3) Calcification and thrombosed part of an aneurysm and its relationship to adjacent structures can be more obviously illustrated.

Sensitivity and specificity of CTA for detecting moderate/severe stenosis deserve our attention. Noticeably, there are two other recent studies by Bash et al. [7], as well, by Nguyen-Huynh et al. [8] indicate some clues of sensitivity and specificity of CTA for detecting moderate/severe stenosis.

It is noted that CTA for detecting moderate/severe stenosis is greater than 97%, as far as for occlusion, given the sensitivity and specificity were even higher (approaching 100%). [6, 7] The positive predictive value of CTA for diagnosing intracranial occlusion was 100% in these studies. Both of these studies evaluated images obtained on earlier generation CT scanners (single- and 4-slice in one study, 8- and 16 slice in the other). The longer image acquisition time in these studies may help to explain the lack of any false-positive findings of occlusion. However, with increased availability and adoption of very fast CT scanning with 64-slice scanners, the improvement is even more.

SECTION 3

Comparison between Two Studies on Sensitivity and Specificity of CTA

Different studies reveal that the positive predictive value of CTA for diagnosing intracranial occlusion was 100%. Sensitivity of CTA for detecting moderate/severe stenosis is >97% while specificity of CTA for detecting moderate/severe stenosis is >97% (See Table 1) [6, 7].

For an interim cocnclusion, the sensitivity and specificity are even higher (approaching 100%) for diagnosing intracranial artery conclusion. The positive predictive value of CTA for diagnosing intracranial artery conclusion is 100% in these studies. [6, 7]

Table 1. Comparison between two studies on *Sensitivity and specificity of CTA*

Different studies	Bash et al.	Nguyen et al.
	The positive predictive value of CTA for diagnosing intracranial occlusion was 100%	The positive predictive value of CTA for diagnosing intracranial occlusion was 100%
	Sensitivity and of CTA for detecting moderate/severe stenosis (>97%);	Specificity of CTA for detecting moderate/severe stenosis (>97%);
	for occlusion, the sensitivity and specificity were even higher (approaching 100%).	for occlusion, specificity were even higher (approaching 100%).
	The positive predictive value of CTA for diagnosing intracranial occlusion was 100% in these studies	The positive predictive value of CTA for diagnosing intracranial occlusion was 100% in these studies

SECTION 4

Comparing Between CAT and DSA

Anderson et al. in 1997 compared computed tomographic angiography (CTA) with selective digital subtraction angiography (DSA) in the discovery of intracranial aneurysms, particularly in the setting of acute SAH. [8]

The authors employed a blinded prospective study with forty patients of known or suspected intracranial saccular aneurysms accepted both CTA and DSA, including thirty two consecutive patients with SAH in whom CTA was carried out after CT images were available as diagnostic for SAH. The interpretation of those CT angiograms was able to confirm the presence, location, and size of the aneurysms, and anatomic characteristics. The information of the number of aneurysm lobes, aneurysm neck size (not greater than 4 mm), and the number of surronding arterial branches were, as well, evaluated. The comparison was then carried out between images obtained with CTA and those obtained with DSA, with the latter images providing as controls. As a result, they found that DSA revealed forty-three aneurysms in thirty patients and excluded intracranial aneurysms in the remaining ten patients. [8]

Table 2. Comparing between CAT and DSA.

the aneurysm-presence alone	sensitivity CTA 86%	specificity 90%
For the presence of an aneurysm	FALSE NEGATIVE IN 6 ANEURYSMS	CAUSES OF FALSE NEGATIVE : 1] technical problems with the image, 2] the minute sized aneurysm domes, (for example, 3] the dome sized less than 3 mm), and 4] unusual aneurysm locations (for example

Nevertheless, for the sake of completeness, this author do agree with the disadvantage of CTA as following: CT angiography may fail to illustrate small but important blood vessels e. g. posterior communicating, anterior choroidal, and orbitofrontal arteries.

Both clinicians and neuroradiologists should all be aware of the limitations of CTA and try to minimize any potential Interpretation errors.

As to the aneurysm-presence alone, the sensitivity and specificity for CTA was 86 and 90%, respectively. For the presence of an aneurysm, six CTA showed false negative results and there was only one CT angiogram showed a false positive result. False negative results were usually created by technical problems with the image, the minute sized aneurysm domes, (for an example, the dome sized less than 3 mm), and unusual aneurysm locations (for example, PICA: posterior inferior cerebellar artery aneurysms or intracaversnous carotid aneurysms).

In fact, there has been increasing reliance on CTA and MRA for evaluation of the intracranial vasculature in patients suspected of acute stroke. While DSA traditionally is the gold standard, it is invasive but it is associated with potential complications. Furthermore, DSA is not readily accessible any time day or night. In the acute stroke setting, DSA is typically reserved for

Neurodiagnostic Pitfalls of CT Scans ...

159

patients undergoing therapeutic intervention with intra-arterial thrombolysis or embolectomy.

For instance, Anderson et al.'s result obtained with CTA was then compared with their own results obtained with DSA. In their result, there is more than 95% accurate in determining dome and neck size of aneurysm, aneurysm lobularity, and the presence and number of adjacent arterial branches. [9]

Table 3. Anderson et al's study

Anderson et al. 's result obtained with CTA	compared with the results they obtained with DSA	Accuracy is > 95% in in determining : 1]dome and neck size of aneurysm, 2]aneurysm lobularity, and 3]the presence and 4]number of adjacent arterial branches.
The combination of CTA and DSA	providing a 3-dimensional information of the aneurysmal pathology	

Additionally, CTA/ DSA provides a three-dimensional information of aneurysmal pathology, which has been viewed very helpful for neurosurgical planning. CTA is practical for speedy and comparatively noninvasive uncovering of aneurysms in ordinary locations. In clinical cases of SAH wherein the non-amplified CT and CTA outcome designate a obvious basis of hemorrhage and grant sufficient anatomical features, it is likely to do without DSA prior to an early on vital aneurysm surgery, e. g., a surgery of Posterior Communicating Artery Aneurysm (Pcom). In all other cases, DSA is subsequently indicated.

Hence, it appears to be reasonable to conclude that CTA can complement traditional catheter angiography with its better demonstration of the 3-dimensional anatomy. It can, as well, supply surgical information about the neck, calcification and thrombosed portion of an aneurysm and its relationship to the surrounding anatomical structure.

Nevertheless, we all have to pay attention to the failure of CTA in clearly demonstrating small but important blood vessels such as posterior communicating, anterior choroidal and orbitofrontal arteries. It is vital to realize limitations of CTA in order to minimize any potential interpretation error.

SECTION 5

Comparing Between CTA and Catheterized Cerebral Angiography

Ng et al. (2007) reported that from October 1994 to April 1996, they had 26 patients with 30 proven intracranial aneurysms underwent neurosurgery, the comparison between CTA and catheterized cerebral angiography is as following [6]:

Table 4. Ng et al's study 26 patients with 30 surgical proven intracranial aneurysms

Ng et al. (2007)	October 1994 through April 1996	26 patients with 30 surgical proven intracranial aneurysms underwent neurosurgery, the comparison between CTA and catheterized cerebral angiography is as following : CTA angiography was superior due to following:
		1]illustrating the aneurysmal neck in seven aneurysms,
		2] illustrating the aneurysmal neck in seven aneurysms,
		3] illustrating the aneurysmal neck in seven aneurysms,
		4] was inferior in one.
		5] the thrombosed part and the calcification of aneurysms were obviously better illustrated on CTA. 5] CTA is helpful in distinguishing tight blood vessel loops from aneurysms.
		6] On CTA, one posterior communicating arterial aneurysm was missed and another anterior choroidal artery aneurysm was misinterpreted as a posterior communicating artery aneurysm.

Noticeably, their other two patients in whom the infundibulum of the orbitofrontal artery was misinterpreted on CTA as an anterior communicating artery aneurysm. [6]

SECTION 6

TOF-MRA with its Relationship to a Virtual Reality Environment for *Neurosurgical* Planning

Time-of-flight magnetic resonance angiography (TOF-MRA) is dependent on the flow and the movement of protons in blood through the imaging plane. To accomplish this, the technique involves saturating a signal in the slice that is to be imaged with rapid RF (Radiofrequency) pulses. The RFpulse will suppress background or stationary tissues, whereas fresh-moving blood entering the slice after the RF pulse will retain its signal intensity and create contrast between blood and background tissue. To decrease the time flowing blood spends in the selected slice, slices are chosen perpendicular to blood flow, and often acquisition is coordinated with systolic flow using pulse or electrocardiographic gating. Overestimation of stenosis may take place if blood is flowing parallel to the slice of interest because flowing blood can be inadvertently suppressed. This artifact is often encountered in the foot, and in the region proximal anterior tibial artery. In fact, TOF imaging may be used for arterial or venous imaging. A saturation band may be placed above or below the slice relevant to eradicate flow from artery or veins as wanted. On behalf of peripheral MRA, saturating a slice distal to the imaging slice in order that venous blood is drenched at what time it arrives the imaging slice can ban venous augmentation. [7] Such as, two-dimensional TOF-MRA of the carotid and vertebral arteries will requires the source data obtained in the axial plane, as well as a coronal oblique utmost strength projection image of a normal left carotid bifurcation is on the right. TOF-MRA is then thwarted by flow voids or by low signal strength regions inside blood vessels. Flow voids can arise from in-plane saturation, which takes place while a blood vessel passes in the same plane as the imaging slice, hence, saturating the aortic blood, and, as well, by post-stenotic turbulence distal to a site of stenosis, which in turn intensifies the phase dispersal. [10] TOF-MRA can, as well, amplify the length of occlusion and stenosis of blood vessels [11]

Another issue with TOF-MRA is its rather long imaging times (minutes to hours up to the distance covered and patient's degree of cooperation) due to the need of saturation pulses directing the imaging slice perpendicular to the blood flow. [7] On the other hand, with parallel imaging techniques, which is an innovative way of filling k-space, imaging time can be reduced as in this technique - a special RF receiver coils. In fact, TOF-MRA may be carried out by using two to three dimensional techniques and is still used as a vital portion

162 Bing H Tang and Eve Tiu

of neurovascular imaging due to the fact that it is quite perceptive to flow, especially the blood flow, and can be carried out with rather great deal of resolution. Just like other MRA techniques, TOF-MRA is sensitive to relics that are due to metallic effects and other devices in the neighborhood.

Noticeably, as a result of clinical necessity, sometimes patients have to receive intravenous tissue plasminogen activator (tPA) prior to undergoing 3-dimensional (TOF) intracranial MRA. [9]. With regard to tPA and Thrombolysis, see the reference of [1] and vide supra SECTION 1.

After thrombolysis, there often are more radiological studies such as MRA and DSA can be done for further evaluation of the same patients on the same day. For example, on CTA alone before Thrombolysis using tPA, one may initially find occlusion of basilar artery as well as occlusion of bilateral distal vertebral arteries. Nonetheless, after thrombolysis, a delayed contrast-augumented CT may subsequently illustrate a smooth flow of the distal vertebral and entire basilar artery. One explanation for such a contradiction is that such a patient's basilar artery might be thrombosed between the time of CTA and MRA/DSA. The absence of any neurological deficits found between examinations at two different points in time, as would be anticipated with a characteristically tempting basilar artery occlusion, one should consider against this radiological risk. [10, 15] A more probable clarification for this radiological contradiction lies in the fact that various imaging modalities differ in ways of capturing and assessing vascular flow.

For a summary of the aforementioned discussion thus far, performing CTA, MRA and DSA without pitfalls of interpretation errors require sound understanding of both the technical parameters and early recognition of potential technical artifacts underlying each diagnostic modality.

SECTION 6

CTA for Diagnosis of Carotid Artery Stenosis/Occlusion

Three-dimensional intracranial TOF-MRA shows from equivalent to slightly lower sensitivity of MRA as compared with CTA for diagnosis of carotid artery stenosis-occlusive disease. Sensitivity ranges between 70% and 100% for detecting moderate/severe stenosis, and between 87% and 100% for occlusion; conversely, specificity is close to 100% for both. [7, 8, 9]

Table 5. CTA for diagnosis of carotid artery

CTA for diagnosis of carotid artery	Sensitivity ranges	Spefificity
detecting moderate/severe stenosis	between 70% to 100%	almost 100%
detecting for occlusion	between 87% to 100%	almost 100%

CTA for diagnosis of carotid artery

SECTION 7

MR Angiography (MRA) AND ITS FUNCTION

MRA has several important limitations. Unlike CTA and DSA, which employ a contrast agent to directly image the blood flow within a vessel, TOF MRA largely relies on the magnetization of spins flowing into an imaging slice and is prone to certain flow artifacts.

As TOF-MRA useing a gradient echo series and a swift progression of radiofrequency to put down the lid of signal from the motionless backdrop body-tissue, hence blood positioned beyond the imaging plane stays comparatively undistracted by the pulses, and flows into the imaging plane with magnetization undamaged, thus generates clear MR signal (flow-associated augmentation). By itself, perfect TOF imaging entails that backdrop of human body tissue to be totally concealed, and that inward bound blood to be absolutely unsaturated to engender maximal signal. This is not practically for all time attainable.

Since latent drawbacks is significant for accurate interpretation of MRA, indeed radiologically speaking, backdrop may not be entirely inhibited with tissues in human body, such as fat, blood such as SAH, and/or tissue swelling such as CE or blood clot such as ICH, IVH, EPH and SDH etc. These physiological or pathological tissues may rapidly recover their longitudinal magnetization in spite of the hasty succession of RF pulses, and are able to engender obvious MR signal that may get in the way with image interpretation and hence may be difficult to understand the true nature of blood vessels, especially arteries.

On the other hand, smooth blood flow, to the contrary, may also feel saturation influences by RF pulses. Slow flowing blood takes more time inside a set imaging volume, creating it to be susceptible to penetration by RF pulses. Regions of slow flow because of previous or latter stenosis/thrombosis may have signal disappearance and the blood vessels thus look like occluded.

Hence, in regions of unstable blood flow near a stenotic site can, as well, look like occluded because of signal loss. The surveillance of signal disappearance because of spin dephasing at the site of stenoses with turbulent flow has been pictured in both phantom models and biomedical researches. [6, 8, 9]. As a matter of fact, in cases of vessel occlusion that may not be detected, TOF imaging frequently uses a saturation band to subdue all flow-involved enhancement contradictory in direction to arterial flow, when it comes down to it, characteristically deletes unwelcome venous signal but may, as well, have the accidental outcome of inhibiting retrospective collateral blood flow.

SECTION 8

A Comparison of Positive Predictive Values between CTA and MRA in Bash et al's Cases

Table 6. A Comparison of positive predictive values between CTA and MRA in Bash et al. al's cases

CTA	MRA	Remark
For acute cerebrovascular events, positive predictive values of 93% for stenosis	For acute cerebrovascular events positive predictive values of 65% for stenosis	
positive predictive values of 100% for occlusion	positive predictive values of 59% for occlusion	
For basilar artery patent in CTA when the complete absence of any clinical deterioration noted	For the impression of basilar artery occlusion in MRA when the complete absence of any clinical deterioration noted, then MRA in such an instance was falsely positive for occlusion.	Be aware of the fact that an sound understanding of the fact is important as following : the flow artifacts are common to TOF MRA.

Bash et al. al compared CTA, MRA and DSA findings in patients suspected of acute cerebrovascular events, and found that MRA had positive

Neurodiagnostic Pitfalls of CT Scans ...

predictive values of 65% for stenosis and 59% for occlusion, compared with 93% and 100% for CTA. [7]

Known the possibility for relic signal disappearance with TOF MRA in cases of distorted flow, it is unsurprising that MRA has a greater false-positive rate for discovery of intracranial stenosis and blood vessel occlusion. Adequate knowledge of the aforementioned latent drawbacks is significant for accurate interpretation of MRA. This is particularly pertinent to acute stroke imaging, since most patients with cerebral thromboembolic disease are more probable to have modifications in flow movement and action with delayed and disturbed flow, including but not limited to turbulent flow and disturbing retrograde flow.

SECTION 9

Digital Subtraction Angiography (DSA)

DSA is traditionally considered as the gold standard for assessment of the intracranial vasculature, and is the modality with which CTA and MRA are compared. In some cases, perhaps DSA showed occlusion of most of basilar artery, with only minimal opacification of the vertebrobasilar confluence and basilar tip (the latter via posterior communicating arteries on carotid injection). However, CTA and delayed contrast-enhanced CT had previously shown good opacification of the basilar artery and there had been no interval change in the patient's clinical status during the time interval between CT and DSA.

Under such a circumstance, known the CT finding with stable clinical examination, it is likely that DSA reflected a false-positive finding of basilar artery occlusion. Bash et al. reported cases of false-positive DSA findings of occlusion in 6 of 28 patients (21%) who presented with symptomatology of acute stroke and underwent CTA, MRA and DSA.

Table 7.

28 patients	6 patients		all 6 patients undergone all 3 test methods	all 6 patients MRA	
				True positive	False positive
	6	21%		4 patients	2 patients

Hence, it appears that cerebral blood circulation took place in very slow-flow or low-flow states distal to a significant stenosis, which may cause the vessel to appear occluded on DSA. MRA was, as well, falsely positive for occlusion in 4 of those 6 cases that Bash et al. reported. The conclusion of a false-positive DSA finding was then reached by consensus re-assessment of the data in all aforementioned six cases.

Hence, it has become obvious that in CTA and DSA findings in Bash et al's cases [7], as well, in other reported cases, lies in differences in image acquisition time. Angiographic runs are characteristically attained over 5 sec (at a rate of 4 frames-per-second film) and held a single intracranial circulation cycle.

Table 8. A 64-slice CTA A single intracranial circulation cycle (According to   and   .).rr to check

A single intracranial circulation cycle		
	is counting from opacification of the carotid siphon	to maximal opacification of the cerebral cortical veins
A 64-slice CTA is extraordinarily speedy		
	As comparing with the time needed from the injection of contrast material to the time of scan ending, ranges about from 20 to 25 sec, as well, it keeps more time for contrast material circulating through regions of extensive stenosis;	Delayed contrast-augumented CT attained 60 sec after CTA provides more time for contrast material circulating to opacify patent segments of the blood vessel lumen on either side of stenotic/occluded regio
	Such a velocity of CTA is faster than that of DSA.	

Normally speaking, a single intracranial circulation cycle is counting from opacification of the carotid siphon to maximal opacification of the cerebral cortical veins, takes about 4 to 6 sec. [12, 13]

Obviously, literature-review highlights significant meanings about intracranial blood vessel imaging with CTA, MRA and DSA. Indeed CTA and MRA have quite fairly high sensitivity/specificity for revealing intracranial stenoses and occlusions, while using DSA as the gold standard. Nonetheless, blood flow combining the contrast material flow create certain extent of artifacts, which can result in the look of blood vessel occlusion in respective modality, though the mechanism involved varies.

SECTION 10

Signal Loss in TOF MRA

It has been well recognized that Signal Loss can take place because of sluggish, turbulent or back flow. On the contrary, flow-associated artifacts are not characteristically related with CTA or DSA. When acquisition times turn out to be even shorter in any scanners with greater–detector-row CT, the likelihood of image acquisition going beyond the contrast material bolus, and then resulting in types of pseudo-occlusion ought to be seriously assessed. [7]

A sound and full understanding of these latent drawbacks is helpful and may avoid imprecise explanation of imaging result raised by movement and action change of blood flow in patients with cerebral blood vessel disease.

SECTION 11

Drawbacks and Mistakes of CT Angiography (CTA)

Takhtani D et al. addressed more than a few drawbacks and mistakes of CTA with graphic demonstration and means to conquer future misinterpretations. As CTA has increasingly been employed for the noninvasive evaluation of the carintracraneal carotid and intracranial vessels. Ease of data attainment may contradict the complexity of interpreting each individual vessel as well as may affect the extent of correctly understanding countless post-processing techniques. Hence, diagnostic harvest and precision of CTA are augmented by good data attainment and by full and sound knowledge and completely taking advantage of post-processing techniques [14]. For instance, known the medical notion of cerebral posterior-circulation ischemia, generally speaking, a CT/CTA was ordered and then carried out within the first hour of symptom onset of stroke symptomatology. The ordinary CT stroke protocol should include 64-slice CTA from the base of the heart through the cerebral vertex; as well, a belated contrast-material-enhanced cerebral CT was then obtained approximately 1 min after CTA (without the need for any extra contrast material because contrast material has already been injected for CTA.

Sometimes, one might find that the original CTA illustrated an absence of opacification of the bilateral distal vertebral arteries and proximal basilar artery, while the delayed contrast-enhanced images illustrated customary opacification of the distal vertebral artery and proximal basilar artery. As a matter of fact, Kim et al. once illustrated the absence of flow-associated augumented in the bilateral distal vertebral and the whole basilar artery, which were different from the initial CTA's finding. The authors' attention was paid particularly to the precaution of being no change in the patient's clinical examination, as well as, no evidence of neurologic deterioration between initial CTA and the follow-up MRA either. The patient then undertook DSA the ensuing day, approximately 24 hours after the original CTA, to reevaluate the patient's blood vessel condition. There was no neurological deterioration during the time of those follow-up diagnostic tests. DSA at that juncture illustrated occlusion of the right vertebral artery, as well, occlusion of the left vertebral artery just proximal to the posterior inferior cerebellar artery (PICA); reconstitution of the vertebrobasilar confluence distal to PICA was then carried out, with successful release of occasion of the remainder of the basilar artery. [15]

SECTION 12

179 Consecutive Patients with Spur-of-the-Moment SAH, During a Period Over 36 Months, as Detected by Viewing CT and CTA

Prestigiacomo C et al. last year reported 179 consecutive patients with spur-of-the-moment SAH, during a period over 36 months, as detected by viewing CT and CTA. Patients with negative CTA findings undertook DSA within 24 hours of the initial episode. All patients who were initially diagnosed to have angiographically negative finding for SAH undertook

Neurodiagnostic Pitfalls of CT Scans ... 169

follow-up DSA two weeks later. Hence the authors conclude that sensitivity and specificity were higher than previously reported in literature, suggesting that CTA may be used as an initial screening tool instead of DSA. Further studies are necessary to determine if CTA can supplant DSA in ruling out all types of cerebral vascular disease in idiopathic SAH. [16]

The noise power spectrum (NPS) is the orientation metric for appreciating the noise component in computed tomography (CT) images. In order to assess the noise natures of clinical multidetector (MDCT) scanners, local 2D and 3D NPSs were calculated for various attainment reconstruction parameters.

Table 9. Prestigiacomo et al. reported 179 consecutive patients with spur-of-the-moment SAH during a period over 36 months, as detected by viewing CT and CTA. Patients with negative CTA findings undertook DSA within 24 hours of arrangement. All patients who were clinically diagnosed to have angiographically negative SAH undertook follow-up DSA two weeks later. Among those 179 patients checked by CTA, as the following tabulatio

Prestigiacomo et al. reported 179 patients checked by:		
	CTA	MRI
	13 (7%) were negative for aneurysms, arteriovenous malformation or dural fistula on CTA.	The MRI taken in order to exclude thrombosed aneurysms and the repeated angiography at the 2 week interval for follow-up were negative Those 13 patients were then undertook DSA. There was no new lesions detected on six-vessel-angiography,
	Hence CAT : 1] None false negative rate	
	2] sensitivity 100%, 3] predictive value 100%	

SECTION 13

Three Dimensional Noise Power Spectrum Applied on Clinical MDCT Scanners: Effects of Reconstruction Algorithms and Reconstruction Filters

For example, a 64- and a 128-MDCT scanners were employed. Measurements were carried out on a water phantom in axial and helical attainment modes. For both installations, CT dose index was identical. The effects of parameters were researched for but not limiting to the following important items: the reconstruction filter (soft, standard and bone) and the reconstruction algorithm (filtered-back projection (FBP), adaptive statistical iterative reconstruction (ASIR)) were investigated. Images were then reconstructed in the coronal plane using a reformat process.

Subsequently, 2D and 3D NPS methods were calculated. In axial attainment mode, the 2D axial NPS revealed essential scale dissimilarity as a function of the z-direction when gauged at the phantom center. On the other hand, in helical mode, a directional reliance with lobular figure was scrutinized at the same time as the scale of the NPS was reserved steady. Significant influences of the reconstruction filter, pitch and reconstruction algorithm were scrutinized on 3D NPS results for both MDCTs.

In fact, with ASIR, a reduction of the NPS scale and a change of the NPS peak to the low frequency scope can be viewed. The two dimensional coronal NPS attained from the reformat images was impact ed by the exclamation while compared to 2D coronal NPS obtained from 3D capacity. The noise nature of volume checked in last generation MDCTs was researched employing local 3D NPS metric. Nonetheless, the influence of the movable noise effect may require further studies. [17]

CONCLUSION

This chapter might be a so-called caricature presentation of the genuine and complex neororadiological pitfalls' review, though it is merely a personal perspective. A lot is still remained to be discovered. For instances, Primary Fibrinolytic Syndrome, NPS as the orientation metric for appreciating the noise component in CT images, and 3D noise power spectrum applied on clinical MDCT scanner, as well, some more others are in need of further study.

REFERENCES

[1] Tang B., McKenna P., Rovit R. Primary Fibrinolytic Syndrome Associated with Subarachnoid Hemorrhage. *Angiology*, Nov. 1973, 627-34

[2] Tang B. Disseminated Intravascular Coagulation. In Chiu Wen-da ed. *Recent Advances in Neurotraumatology*, first edition, Italy, Monduzzi Editore, Nov 20, 1999: 137—43

[3] Sherry, S. Fibrinolysis, Annual Review of Medicine, Vol.19: 247, Edited by Graff, A.C. and Creger, W.P., Palo Alto. *Annual Reviews Inc.*,1968.

[4] Back, N. and Ambrus, J.L.: *Fibrinolysis, Surgical Bleeding, a Handbook for Medicine, Surgery and Specialties*, p.390, edited by Ulin, A.W. and Golub, S., 1966.

[5] Tang, B. The critical analysis on diagnosis of Disseminated Intravascular Coagulation with Screening Tests-a Scoring System and Related Literature Review. *JAMC* Oct-Dec 2007; 19(4):112-120

[6] Ng Shu-Hang, Ho-Fai Wongb, Sheung-Fat Kob, Chi-Ming Leeb, Pao-Sheng Yenb, Yau-Yau Waib and Yung-Liang Wang. *CT angiography of intracranial aneurysms: advantages and pitfalls*. 1997.

[7] Bash S, Villablanca JP, Jahan R, et al. Intracranial vascular stenosis and occlusive disease: Evaluation with CT angiography, MR angiography, and digital subtraction angiography. **AJNR Am J Neuroradiol. ** 2005;26:1012-1021.

[8] Nguyen-Huynh MN, Wintermark M, English J, et al. How accurate is CT angiography in evaluating intracranial atherosclerotic disease? *Stroke.* 2008; 39:1184-1188.

[9] Anderson, Glenn B. ; Findlay, J. Max ; Steinke, David E. ; Ashforth Robert. Experience with Computed Tomographic Angiography for the Detection of Intracranial Aneurysms in the Setting of Acute Subarachnoid Hemorrhage. *Neurosurgery* September 1997 - Volume 41 - Issue 3 - pp 522-528

[10] Korogi Y,Takahashi M, Nakagawa T, et al. Intracranial vascular stenosis and occlusion: MR angiographic findings. **AJNR Am J Neuroradiol.* *1997;18:135-143.

[11] Bradley WG, Jr., Waluch V, Lai KS, et al. The appearance of rapidly flowing blood on magnetic resonance images. *AJR Am J Roentgenol.* *1984; 143:1167-1174.

[12] Greitz T.A radiologic study of the brain circulation by rapid serial Gngiography of the carotid artery. *Acta Radiol Suppl.* *1956:1-123.

[13] Milburn JM, Moran CJ, Cross DT, 3rd, et al. Effect of intraarterial papaverine on cerebral circulation time. *AJNR Am J Neuroradiol.* *1997;18: 1081-1085. *Applied Radiology*

[14] Takhtani D. Anterior subtemporal approach for posteriorly projecting posterior. *J. of American Roentgen Ray Society.*

[15] Kim, J, and Max Wintermark, MD Volume 39, Number 04, April 2010. Intracranial vascular imaging: *Pearls and pitfalls Jane*

[16] Prestigiacomo C et al. last year (2010) J NeuroIntervent Surg 2010,2:385-389 Intracranial vascular imaging: *Pearls and pitfalls*

[17] Fredéric A. Miéville, Gregory Bolard, Mohamed Benkreira, Paul Ayestaran, François Gudinchet, François Bochud and Francis R. Verdun, "3D noise power spectrum applied on clinical MDCT scanners: effects of reconstruction algorithms and reconstruction"

In: CT Scans
Editors: V. E. Perkel et al.

ISBN 978-1-62100-319-9
©2012 Nova Science Publishers, Inc.

Chapter 5

3D-CT IN ORAL AND MAXILLOFACIAL RESEARCH

R. M. Yáñez-Vico, D. Torres-Lagares, A. Iglesias-Linares, D. González-Padilla, E. Solano-Reina and J. L. Gutierrez-Pérez

Departamento de Estamologia, Facultad de Odontologia, Universidad de Sevilla, Spain

ABSTRACT

The arrival of the digital image to the oral and maxillofacial world has led to new research fields arising which are focused on the diagnostic potential of image manipulation in radiography. Many of those proposals have resulted in valuable tools that increase the diagnostic utility. However, many digital images have the same limitations as those found in conventional cephalometric analyses including magnification, distortion and superimposition of anatomical structures.

The analysis of the craniofacial complex has improved recently with the development of three-dimensional image technology, since we are able to observe any one of the craniofacial bones from different angles using the three-dimensional images obtained from computed tomography. Technology using 3D image provides a very effective tool for evaluating, characterizing, and drawing up the surgical treatment plan for potential orthognathic surgery patients.

An important advancement in computed tomography (CT) technology came thanks to Herman and Liu. In 1977, who presented three-dimensional reconstructions from axial slides. This method meant that it was no longer necessary to create mental three-dimensional images from two-dimensional data (those from conventional X-ray machines and from axial CT scanners), which is often inaccurate or even impossible.

The CT enables us to ascertain an exact image of the anatomical structures in three dimensions and to visualize both the soft tissues and the skeletal structures in 3D, thus improving the preparatory planning of many surgical procedures.

A new generation of compact CT scanners has been developed, specially designed for use in the head and neck region. These ultra-compact CT scanners employ cone beam geometry (cone beam - CBCT) which uses X-ray photons much more efficiently. The x-ray dose is lower in the CBCT and conventional images such as panoramic, lateral and anterior/posterior radiographs can be obtained from it. Nevertheless, three-dimensional images mean new changes and they must be interpreted in a new different way in order to extract the most information possible for the diagnosis, planning and simulation of the treatment.

INTRODUCTION

The conventional imaging methods do not provide consistent accurate results and therefore, alternative imaging methods for diagnosis need to be developed and studied to potentially improve landmark identification and linear and angular measurements. These precise anatomical data cannot be obtained by any other means but radiological imaging in three dimensions. The craniofacial skeleton can be viewed in three dimensions using computed tomography [1, 2]. It is possible to obtain precise anatomical relationships in three dimensions with CT, which improves the preoperative planning of many surgical procedures [3].

The substitution of conventional cephalometry for cephalometry based on 3D virtual models using CT in order to monitor the craniofacial relationship is potentially an important step forward in the diagnosis and treatment of orthodontic and surgical patients. Many of the limitations associated with conventional X-rays can be reduced; however, 3D data display new changes and require a different approach to that which we are used to in order to obtain as much information as possible.

THREE-DIMENSIONAL COMPUTED TOMOGRAPHY IMAGE VERSUS CONVENTIONAL X-RAY

In the middle of the nineteen eighties, computed tomography was presented to model the structures of the skull in three dimensions for maxillofacial surgery [4]. Computed tomography is an imaging modality that produces cross-sectional planes representing the X-ray attenuation properties of the tissues. The image is formed using an X-ray beam and a series of acquisitions is carried out covering the entire field of view.

This process is repeated for a large number of angles, taking line attenuation measurements for all possible angles and measured distances from the center. Based on all these measurements, the present attenuation of each point of the scanned volume is reconstructed. Attenuated X-rays are captured by the detectors of the scanner and they are digitized. Reconstruction algorithms then create the different layers of the CT. These layers, therefore, have a digital nature. An open communication protocol has been adapted to transmit and communicate these digital layers of the CT, known as DICOM (Digital Imaging and Communications in Medicine) (Figure 1). A conventional CT produces a set of images that represent axial layers and are usually displayed as conventional 2D images.

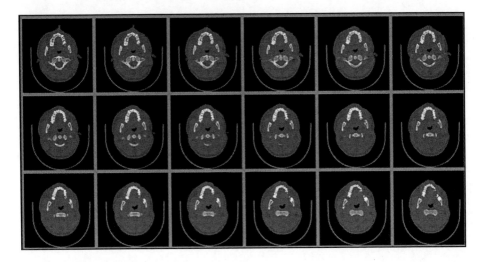

Figure 1. DICOM image.

The main disadvantages of this technique are: high radiation dose; limited resolution of soft tissues due to layer thickness (normally 5 mm); and the presence of metallic objects as there may be amalgam restorations or orthodontic fixed appliances.

In a conventional X-ray, the digitized image is made up of pixels, which are small square elements set out in rows and columns. Each pixel has a value of brightness and color representing the density of the X-ray when it crosses the corresponding structure. Volume is obtained by extending a flat image in the third dimension. The volumetric image is made up of voxels, which are like small buckets, arranged one next to another.

CT volume consists of a 3D matrix of elements called voxels (Figure 2) which usually have a 12-bit number scale, expressed in Hounsfield units (HU). By definition, water normally has 0 HU and air around 1000 HU. In a similar way to the flat images, the values of brightness of each bucket represent the density of the corresponding anatomical structure. This means that the data that we see, for example of the human head, does not come as a layer upon layer, but as one complete structure in 3D that we can move and examine from any angle. Also, we can measure this structure just as in 2D conventional cephalometry and remove the regions that are not of interest.

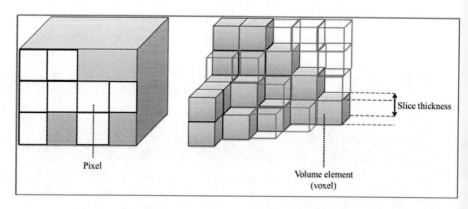

Figure 2. Left: representation of 2D image with pixel elements. Right: representation of 3D image with voxel elements.

Several techniques of CT reconstruction have been used for the diagnosis, planning and simulation of treatment. However, many changes to the superimposition of images should be considered in order to assess the changes produced by the treatment. Landmark identification in a three-dimensional virtual model requires suitable operational definitions of the landmark location in each one of the three planes of the space [5].

Dentists have been using cephalometry for more than 70 years and orthodontists have become used to using lateral X-rays to examine patients and plan treatment. These methods are already very well established and extensive and diverse results have been presented in normal populations as well as in treated patients [6, 7]. Nevertheless, 2D images provide inconsistent information in some patients with deformities [8-10]. The majority of the images that are used to analyze and diagnose anomalies of the craniofacial complex are X-rays, especially lateral and panoramic. For this reason, it is very difficult to be able to distinguish between the different anatomical landmarks of the right and left side. In addition, 2D X-rays have inherent limitations such as the extension and distortion of the image that can lead to a wrong diagnosis. Inherent magnification of the image takes place in the lateral and frontal views depending on the distance of the structure to the film, whereas 3D-CT methods provide an orthogonal image on a scale 1:1. A conventional 2D panoramic view leads to the superimposition of the vertebrae and the contralateral side, and the image in the anterior region is often of poor quality. However, the 3D-CT panoramic view makes it possible to erase irrelevant structures that complicate the physician's view. In addition, it facilitates the identification of the thickness of the alveolar bone, eruption, dental development and its relative position with respect to the dental roots. Facial analysis is also improved using these 3D methods since translucency can be changed and the relationships between soft tissues and bones determined.

Lateral X-rays collapse three-dimensional structure into a bidimensional plane. This usually leads to two types of errors: errors of projection and errors of identification.

The projection errors arise as magnifications are imperfect as a result of the different distances between the center, the objects of interest (landmarks) and the image receptor.

A certain amount of inherent magnification always exists because X-ray photons emanate from the center in a divergent way. The degree of magnification is determined by the relative distances between the X-ray source and the object and the distance between the source and the film. In order to diminish this magnification, the X-ray source must be 1.5 m from the mid-sagittal plane of the head of the patient. This ensures that the X-ray photons travel as parallel as possible through the object, thus, reducing magnification.

Nevertheless, magnification still exists in the majority of oral and craniofacial structures. This magnification oscillates between zero, in objects near to the film and in the exact center of the ray beam cone, and up to 24% in the most distant regions such as the ear plugs. In addition, this magnification is not constant for all the possible sagittal radiographic planes of the patient [11, 12]. As a result, the structures located nearest to the X-ray film will undergo less magnification than those located in the mid-sagittal plane, and these will undergo less magnification than those nearest the X-ray beam. Therefore, if the beam penetrates a patient from right to left, the image of the right side will be larger than the one of the left side (Figure 3) [13].

Moreover, there are also projection errors that are caused by the deviations of the geometry of the standard projection and the incorrect alignment of the cephalostat if the patients' head rotates in any plane [14, 15].

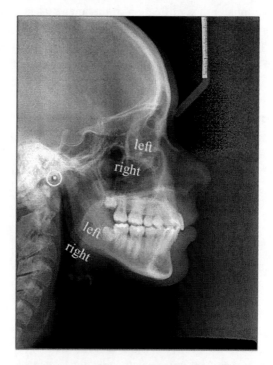

Figure 3. Lateral X-ray which shows the magnification between left and right skeletal structures. The left side of the patient has been positioned close to the X-ray film, so the X-ray beam has penetrated from right to left.

Identification errors are due to variability in locating the different landmarks. Several factors such as the quality of the X-ray image, the precision of the definition of the landmark and the consistency of the location of the landmark as well as operator variability would result in large changes being clearly observed, whereas subtle changes would remain imperceptible [16, 17].

Grummons and Kappeyne van de Copello [18] investigated asymmetry by means of frontal analyses. They found that frontal cephalometric measures were subject to distortion due to the projection technique and that they could not be used for either quantitative or comparative purposes. As quantitative measures are key factors for the diagnosis of asymmetry, an analysis of this type with X-rays films in two dimensions would not be suitable.

Simplified three-dimensional images of facial bones have also been developed by computer using the appropriate coordinate to the anatomical landmarks that can normally be seen in frontal and lateral X-rays [19]. The main problem of this is that it is only possible to use anatomical landmarks that are well defined in both projections. For this reason, a 3D-CT analysis would be indispensable for this type of study.

Rachmiel et al. [20] carried out measurements on coronal images in patients with hemifacial microsomia. These researchers used a horizontal plane at the level of the fronto-zygomatic suture, defining a line connecting the bilateral latero-orbitalis and a vertical line perpendicular to the *crista galli*. This way, they mainly evaluated the degree of deviation from the mid-mandibular point, the degree of deviation of the occlusal plane from the horizontal reference line and the difference between the heights of mandibular rami. The main limitations were in identifying the anatomical landmarks in the posterior area of the skull, as they were the *Sella* and the *Basion*, due to the superimposition and darkening of the most anterior anatomical structures. This means that reference planes based on the anatomy of the cranial base would not be used in this type of study.

The development of CT and computer science technology enables us to have easy access to 3D images of the craniofacial complex. Soft tissues, such as those of skeletal structures, can be viewed using CT in the three planes of space [21]. 3D-CT images are accurate enough for linear measurements [22, 23]. Calvanti et al. [23] investigated precision by comparing the results of linear measurements on 3D-CT images with physical measurements performed on dry skulls. They concluded that the difference between the two measurements was minimal and that the images in 3D were very accurate. In recent years, this has improved further with the appearance of helical CT [24]. There are no problems with the superimposition of structures in 3D-CT images and the position of the anatomical landmarks can be defined completely. In addition, the structures can be viewed from any angle. The precision and consistency of this type of image have been confirmed. In studies with helical CT, Matteson et al. [25] and Hildebolt et al. [26] measured the skull using 3D-CT and reported favorable findings.

The use of a precise and reproducible instrument to analyze the images produced by this type of technology provides clinicians with new diagnostic possibilities. In this sense, we want to highlight the evaluation of craniofacial asymmetries, diagnosis and planning of the treatment of patients affected with craniofacial syndromes and candidates for orthognathic surgery amongst the main benefits of conventional cephalometric diagnosis.

3D CEPHALOMETRIC DIAGNOSIS

Since cephalometric X-rays arrived in 1931 [27, 28], this method has been widely used as a descriptive, analytical and diagnostic tool, particularly in Orthodontics and Maxillofacial surgery, in diagnosis and clinical planning of the treatment as well as in research. This technique uses quantitative measurements obtained from landmarks. Craniofacial morphology of the same subjects from growth has been studied over different periods. In addition, it helps orthodontists and surgeons acquire a greater understanding of how growth processes can have an effect on the treatment of patients [29].

From 1931, many studies that investigated the utility and the validity of cephalometry analyses have been published. Cephalometrics is mainly based on the use of lateral X-rays, where the landmarks and measurements are carried out in the mid-sagittal plane. Some studies have provided us with standard measurements of craniofacial variables [30-32]. The landmarks are identified on the film or on the hardcopy of the image. A selection of linear and angular measurements to produce standards for the different ages is then obtained. In addition to this, there is the recent incorporation of computer-assisted technology which makes it possible and easy to compare and evaluate the craniofacial anatomy.

The landmarks used in conventional radiological cephalometry are normally defined manually. Nevertheless, several authors [33, 34] have tried to automatize the tedious process of manual marking. Cephalometric measurements (manual or automatic) are normally analyzed by statistical comparison with measurements from a control group. This process has been applied in the conventional way for the study, for example, of the craniofacial growth in cleft lip and palate patients [35-37], studies of children with diverse malocclusions [38-40] and mandibular growth analysis [41].

Nevertheless, authors such as Ahlqvist et al. [7], Houston et al. [43], Kamoen et al. [44] and Singh et al. [37] have documented numerous disadvantages in the use of this cephalometry. The data are only in two dimensions, and the images can be distorted due to the projection of the three-dimensional objects in two dimensions. Furthermore, the diverse effects of magnification must also be considered. The analysis of the data is limited and frequently inadequate when trying to describe a three-dimensional complex structure such as the skull. It is impossible to identify the majority of three-dimensional craniofacial characteristics in detail in traditional 2D cephalometry. Furthermore, it is necessary to take the measurement errors into account due to the nature of the images. Maue-Dickson [45], in a revision article, highlighted the errors that arose from selecting some landmarks to be interpreted and judge the direction of facial growth. The location of metallic markers in the maxilla as well as in the mandible in growing patients has made it possible to superimpose on presumably stable structures [46]. Nevertheless, a difference between 5 and 7 degrees was found when comparing craniometric methods with the gonial angle measured using lateral X-rays of skull. The difference is statistically significant and it could be attributed to a systematic error in the radiological method, which would lead to the gonial angle being magnified. For that reason, it is necessary to remember that this technique must always be used with caution taking its limitations into consideration.

The concept of 3D cephalometry has been used by orthodontist and maxillofacial surgeons in literature for many years as an analysis based on the three planes of the space (lateral, frontal and transverse) generated by conventional 2D X-rays [18], but these approaches are not true 3D. To our knowledge, Ono et al. [47] were the first to use a CT helical scanner to carry out 3D measurements on the craniofacial skeleton. Later, other authors [48] applied this technology to demonstrate the value of computed tomography to develop 3D cephalometry. They even suggested that conventional 2D cephalometry should be replaced by this as its measurements were extremely accurate.

The development of 3D cephalometry provides very accurate measurements because lengths and angles are defined by landmarks located directly on the virtual 3D cranial bone surface. The use of a three-dimensional analysis by means of computed tomography makes it easier to assess conventional orthodontic patients and identify the skeletal and/or actual dento-alveolar factors that cause the malocclusion. This is achieved by identifying not only the conventional characteristics, but also the actual dimensions in the three planes of space, as well as by tilting, rotating and diverging the skeletal structures, or any possible compensations or aggravating factors in this same sense, which could not be identified by other conventional methods. However, all the possibilities that this technology offers must be focused on a different way. Thus, as they are different from the conventional 2D ones, new landmarks need to be defined to be able to take advantage of all that it offers. The entire craniofacial complex can be analyzed in 3D with the aid of cephalometry (Figure 4), which will surely change our way of thinking about the clinical planning of patients, mainly in those cases combined with orthognathic surgery.

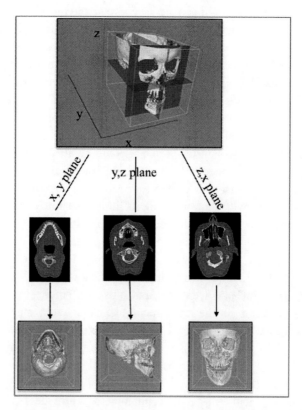

Figure 4. Specific virtual 3D-CT model. It is possible to trace reference planes for 3D cephalometry as seen at the bottom of the image and view any structure from any angle.

Several authors have published their own cephalometries in 3D [49-59], and they emphasize the evaluation of relationships between hard and soft tissues, which is helpful to plan facial esthetics. The use of this technology increases our diagnostic abilities, as we are not solely limited to studying the relationships between the different craniofacial structures. Width of alveolar bone can be assessed in order to evaluate the expansion or inclination movements of teeth, which can then be combined with the axial information of inclination and torque of teeth. Affected teeth can be assessed in the same way. It is possible to identify the exact inclination, angulation and position and their specific relationships to surrounding teeth, which enormously facilitates later surgery as well as the orthodontic mechanics.

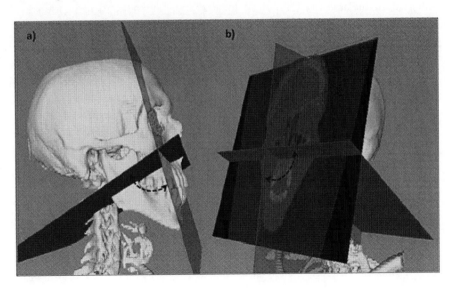

Figure 5. a) Measurement of axial inclination of canines in virtual 3D-CT model. b) Torque of canine measurement in virtual 3D-CT model.

The main limitations of 3D cephalometry are possibly the high cost and the high radiation dose that the patient receives in comparison with conventional 2D cephalometry. In this respect, it is possible to state that we believe that this method is especially useful for patients who need a pre-operative surgical planning and later post-operative evaluations combined with surgical and orthodontic treatment, in which this type of measurement is indicated.

ASYMMETRIC PATIENTS

As we have already described in previous researches [9] craniofacial asymmetry can be diagnosed using conventional X-ray methods, although three-dimensional methods are necessary to carry out a more complete diagnosis.

Posterior-anterior X-ray has become one of the most common clinical X-ray projections to diagnose asymmetry. There are many studies that assess the validity of frontal cephalometry [60, 61]. These studies conclude that there are two basic errors in posterior/anterior projections: those related to the cephalometric method (object-film distance, head rotation) and those that are inherent in the method (landmark localization, landmark identification as a result of the structures' radiolucency, structural superimpositions) [9, 16]. Referring to the head positioning, a simple head rotation would be enough to disturb the perpendicularity of the cranial mid-sagittal line of the X-ray beam leading to distorted measurements. Even if ideal positioning were achieved, it is still especially complicated to locate a proper mid-sagittal axis in patients affected with severe asymmetries. Furthermore, we often consider a proper perpendicular positioning of the connection axis to be between both external auditory holes and the mid-sagittal line, which is usually completely inaccurate. Therefore, asymmetric ears would cause head rotation and therefore, a misinterpretation of the asymmetry [9, 14].

Panoramic X-ray has also been used to assess the asymmetry of the condylar and ramus process and to measure vertical differences between both sides, just as in the methods of Habets et al. [62] or Saglam et al. [63]. However, it is difficult to examine TMJ using radiographs as superimposition of neighboring structures, such as the petrous region of the temporal bone, the mastoid process, and the articular eminence distort and magnify the ramus and the condyle [64]. Although panoramic X-ray technology has an acceptable cost-benefit ratio due to the minimal radiation exposure, the literature does not have great faith in the measurements made with this type of projection [9]. Recently, a systematic review [65] has highlighted once more the poor feasibility of measurements performed on this kind of X-ray and the high variability depending on the X-ray machine.

Submentovertex (SMV) projection provides an excellent view of the cranial base structures enabling the anatomical landmarks on the cranial base to be used to determine the mid-sagittal axis. Despite its inherent benefits, it is used much less in clinical practice than those described above [9].

Williamson et al. [66] studied the identification errors in SMV X-ray. The most significant discrepancy was found in the pogonion (Pg: the most anterior point on the mandible in the mid-sagittal plane of the mandibular symphysis), up to 3.79 mm. Additionally, there was a tendency to superimpose the internal and the external corticals of the frontal region and the dentition on the anterior region of the mandibular symphysis. This superimposition is substantially influenced by head positioning. Lysell et al. [67] suggested that the effects of the projection would be minimal if the mandibular angle were projected immediately anterior to the condyle. The ideal positioning of the head for the SMV radiographies would be when the X-ray beam is perpendicular to the Frankfort plane; however, several limitations exist in patients with reduced mobility of the neck. The intra- and inter-examiner errors were of low reliability in the condylar poles, especially in the vertical direction and in the posterior condylar point of the horizontal direction. Consequently, the authors suggest being cautious when interpreting and using measurements that involve such points due to the high number of errors found with this method [9].

Analyzing the craniofacial complex has improved recently with the development of three-dimensional imaging technology [68], since the three-dimensional images obtained from computed tomography enable us to observe any one of the craniofacial bones from different angles. The etiological structures that cause facial asymmetry can be identified using computed tomography-based 3D models, which is extremely important when planning surgical treatment. Chin deviation may be caused by several factors. We have considered seven possible variations in length as well as angle [69].

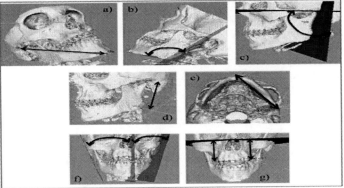

Figure 6. a)Mandibular length; b)Mandibular angle; c)Lateral ramal inclination; d)Ramal height; e)Mandibular body length; f)Frontal ramal inclination; g)Maxillary height

The following can be considered as factors contributing to facial asymmetry (Figure 6): 1)Ramal height: the distance between the highest point of the condyle head (Cdsup) and the lowest point of the gonial region (Goinf; mm); 2)Mandibular body length: the distance between the most posterior point of the gonial region (Gopost) and the lowest point of the mandibular symphysis (Me; mm); 3)Mandibular length: Mandibular length is the distance between Cdsup and Me (mm); 4)Mandibular angle: is defined as the angle formed by the most lateral point of the condyle head and the most lateral point of the gonial region (Cdlat-Golat) with Me-Goinf (°); 5)Maxillary height: from the pulp cavity of the upper first molars (Fmsup) to the Frankfort horizontal plane (Po-Or-Po) (mm); 6)Frontal ramal inclination: Cdlat-Golat to the mid-sagittal reference plane (yz), the angle formed by the mid-sagittal reference plane and the external border of the ramus (°); 7)Lateral ramal inclination: the angle formed by the most posterior points of the condyle head and the gonial region (Cdpost-Gopost) with the Frankfort plane (°).

The previous investigations showed [10] that the structure with the most deviation between the left and right side was the lateral ramal inclination, which was also related directly with asymmetry of the gonion. However, in light of the results, frontal ramal inclination (second most affected structure) seems to be directly related with the appearance of facial asymmetry, if we assume that the chin is the most important factor in determining facial appearance [70]. This should be considered when determining the surgical treatment plan in this type of patient so that they do not present certain noticeable asymmetrical features after the corrective orthodontic-surgical treatment [69]. Other authors [71, 72] have already stated that the assessment of the ramus may influence the choice of surgical treatment. It is important to identify which structures are involved in the appearance of facial asymmetry in subjects who are to undergo orthognathic surgery in order to be able to carry out the correct type of surgery. A reliable diagnosis should be performed for the orthodontic-surgical treatment of patients with facial deformities.

CRANIOFACIAL SYNDROMES: DIAGNOSIS AND ASSESSMENT

Another area of interest for multidisciplinary clinicians is the study of craniofacial syndromes, craniofacial anomalies and cleft lip and palate. Many studies have confirmed how useful 3D-CT can be in growing and developing patients with craniofacial anomalies, since Marsh and Vannier [73] first presented its use in these patients. Darling et al. [64] studied a series of patients with craniosynostosis, fissures of the middle third of the face, trauma and craniofacial syndromes, and they proved the value of 3D-CT compared to 2D-CT. Furthermore, the data found in 3D models could be used to simulate reconstructive surgery for craniofacial abnormalities [74]. For example, Posnick et al. [75] used CT on children with Treacher-Collins zygomatic deficiency. Highly-developed 3D cephalometry is a very useful tool for this type of patient as it offers precise and reliable data of the deficient vectors in the craniofacial structures. It, therefore, makes the vector planning easier in patients who are to undergo bone distraction. Moreover, post-treatment comparisons can be carried out and it is possible to compare how the craniofacial structures grow by using reference planes. Most 3D cephalometries developed use the Saddle point in their reference plane [54-56, 58, 76]. However, the cranial base is deformed in some craniofacial dysmorphisms (e.g. Apert's syndrome), and this may become even more deformed over time. For that reason, an actual representation of craniofacial growth or comparison between forms cannot be obtained by keeping the Saddle point constant. This may distort any change involving this point. For that reason, other points are recommended for the reference plane in the 3D cephalometric system, for example cranial base points, such as foramens, canals and sutures. Some of these have been used as diagnostic indicators for craniofacial dysmorphologies [77, 78].

ORTHOGNATHIC SUGERY

An accurate diagnosis is essential for a correct treatment planning and to provide the patient with the best treatment possible [79]. For that reason, just as in the previous section, three-dimensional models from computed tomography as well as 3D cephalometry are very useful in the diagnosis and planning of candidates for orthognathic surgery, as they are able to analyze the hard and soft tissues of the craniofacial virtual models and their spatial relationship. Three-dimensional computed tomography provides an actual view with exact dimensions of the affected structures in the three planes of space. It, therefore, makes it possible to calculate the structure to be corrected and the direction in which the correction must be made using objective measurements in degrees or millimeters. The tilting of the maxilla or the mandible as well as the frontal ramal inclination is especially significant, and it was practically impossible to obtain this information using conventional cephalometry or conventional planning methods for orthognathic surgery. The models created can be used to simulate the surgical procedure with the different options available and to test them anatomically and esthetically. The soft tissues can be deformed appropriately by moving the hard tissues forward or backward because reconstruction software models tissue properties and attributes that simulate expected changes following treatment [79, 80].

CONCLUSION

The use of computed tomographies represents a substantial improvement in the precision of reproducing skeletal and soft tissue structures. Many techniques have been used in CT reconstruction for the diagnosis, planning and simulation of the treatment. Computed tomographies make possible patient-specific virtual 3D models that provide spatial assessment of the relationships between hard and soft tissues. The use of a precise and consistent instrument to analyze a wide range of images obtained from this kind of technology offers new diagnostic possibilities to clinicians.

The diagnosis of craniofacial asymmetries may be performed using conventional radiographic methods (frontal X-ray, panoramic X-ray and submentovertex X-ray). Such methods have not been found to be very reliable due to inherent projection errors (image magnification, cranial rotation) and identification errors (image quality, precision and reproducibility). Therefore, three-dimensional methods are necessary for a more complete diagnosis. The substitution of conventional X-ray machines for 3D-CT to study craniofacial structures may potentially improve the treatment and diagnosis of orthodontic and orthognathic patients. Many of the limitations of conventional radiographies can be reduced by using 3D technology. However, three-dimensional images require new changes and the they must be interpreted in a different way to which we are used to in order to extract the as much information as possible. New analysis tools are needed to extract, manipulate and synthesize all the diagnostic and therapeutic data in order to interpret them accurately.

REFERENCES

[1] Lascala CA, Panella J, Marques MM. *Analysis of the accuracy of linear measurements obtained by cone beam computed tomography (CBCT-NewTom)*. Dentomaxillofac Radiol 2004; 33:291-4.

[2] Baumrind S, Moffitt F. *Mapping the skull in 3-d.* J Calif Dent Assoc 1972; 48:22-31.

[3] Harrell WE,Jr, Hatcher DC, Bolt RL. *In search of anatomic truth: 3-dimensional digital modeling and the future of orthodontics.* Am J Orthod Dentofacial Orthop 2002;122:325-30.

[4] McCance AM, Moss JP, Fright WR, James DR, Linney AD. *A three dimensional analysis of soft and hard tissue changes following bimaxillary orthognathic surgery in skeletal III patients.* Br J Oral Maxillofac Surg 1992;30:305–12.

[5] Netherway DJ, Abbott AH, Gulamhuseinwala N, McGlaughlin KL, Anderson PJ, *Townsend GC, et al. Three-Dimensional Computed Tomography Cephalometry of Plagiocephaly: Asymmetry and Shape Analysis.* Cleft Palate Craniofac J 2006; 43:201-10.

[6] Richtsmeier JT, Paik CH, Elfert PC, Cole TM, Dahlman HR. *Precision, repeatability, and validation of the localization of cranial landmarks using computed tomography scans.* Cleft Palate Craniofac J 1995;32:217-27.

[7] Ahlqvist J, Eliasson S, Welander U. *The effect of projection errors on cephalometric length measurements.* Eur J Orthod 1986; 8:141-48.

[8] Katusumata A, Fujishita M, Maeda M, Ariji Y, Ariji E, Langlais RO. *3D-CT evaluation of facial asymmetry.* Oral Surg Oral Med Oral Pathol Oral Radiol Endod 2005;99:212-20.

[9] Yañez-Vico RM, Iglesias-Linares A, Torres-Lagares D, Gutiérrez-Pérez JL, Solano-Reina E. *Diagnostic of craniofacial asymmetry.* Literature review. Med Oral Patol Oral Cir Bucal 2010;15:e494-8.

[10] Yáñez-Vico RM, Iglesias-Linares A, Torres-Lagares D, Gutiérrez-Pérez JL, Solano-Reina E. *Three-dimensional evaluation of craniofacial asymmetry: an analysis using computed tomography.* Clin Oral Invest 2010 Jul 15.

[11] Dibbets JM, Nolte K. *Effect of magnification on lateral cephalometric studies.* Am J Orthod Dentofacial Orthop 2002;122:196-201.

[12] Bergensen EO. *Enlargement and distortion in cephalometric radiography: compensation tables for linear measurements.* Angle Orthod 1980;50:230-44.

190   R. M. Yáñez-Vico, D. Torres-Lagares, A. Iglesias-Linares et al.

[13] Chen YJ, Chen SK, Chang HF, Chen KC. *Comparison of landmark identification in traditional versus computer-aided digital cephalometry.* Angle Orthod 2000;70:387-92.

[14] Chen YJ, Chen SK, Huang HW, Yao CC, Chang HF. *Reliability of landmark identification in cephalometric radiography acquired by a storage phosphor imaging system.* Dentomaxillofac Radiol 2004;33:301-6.

[15] Mah J, Hatcher D. *Current status and future needs in craniofacial imaging.* Orthod Craniofac Res 2003; 6 Suppl 1:10-6; discussion 179-82.

[16] Cavalcanti MG, Rocha SS, Vannier MW. *Craniofacial measurements based on 3D-CT volume rendering: implications for clinical applications.* Dentomaxillofac Radiol 2004;33:170-6.

[17] Ekestubbe A, Thilander A, Grondahl K, Grondahl HG. *Absorbed doses from computed tomography for dental implant surgery: comparison with conventional tomography.* Dentomaxillofac Radiol 1993;22:13-7.

[18] Grummons DC, Kappeyne van de Coppello MA. *A frontal asymmetry analysis.* J Clin Orthod 1987;21:448-65.

[19] Kusnoto B, Figueroa AA, Polley JW. *A longitudinal threedimentional evaluation of the growth pattern in hemifacial microsomia treated by mandibular distraction osteogenesis: a preliminary report.* J Craniofac Surg 1999;10:480-6.

[20] Rachmiel A, Manor R, Peled M, Laufer D. *Intraoral distraction osteogenesis of the mandible in hemifacial microsoma.* J Oral Maxillofac Surg 2001;59:728-33.

[21] Xia J, Ip HH, Samman N, Wang D, Kot CS, Yeung RW, et al. *Computer-assisted three-dimensional surgical planning and simulation: 3D virtual osteotomy.* Int J Oral Maxillofac Surg 2000;29:11-7.

[22] Christiansen EL, Thompson JR, Kopp S. *Intra- and inter-observer variability and accuracy in the determination of linear and angular measurements in computed tomography.* An in vitro and in situ study of human mandibles. Acta Odontol Scand 1986;44:221-9.

[23] Cavalcanti MG, Haller JW, Vannier MW. *Three-dimensional computed tomography landmark measurement in craniofacial surgical planning: experimental validation in vitro.* J Oral Maxillofac Surg 1999;57:690-4.

[24] Kawamata A, Ariji Y, Langlais RP. *Three-dimensional computed tomography imaging in dentistry.* Dent Clin North Am 2000;44:395-410.

3D-CT in Oral and Maxillofacial Research   191

[25] Matteson SR, Bechtold W, Phillips C. *A method for threedimensional image reformation for quantitative cephalometric analysis.* J Oral Maxillofac Surg 1989;47:1053-61.

[26] Hildebolt CF, Vannier MW, Knapp RH. *Validation study of skull three-dimensional computerized tomography measurements.* Am J Phys Anthropol 1990;82:283-94.

[27] Broadbent B. *A new x-ray technique and its application to orthodontia.* Angle Orthod 1931;1:45-66.

[28] Hofrath H. *Die bedeutung der rontgenfern und abstandsaufnahme fur die diagnostik der keiferanomalien.* Fortschr Ortho 1931;1:232-42.

[29] Kreiborg S. *Crouzon Syndrome – A Clinical and Roentgencephalometric Study (Doctorate thesis).* Copenhagen: Institute of Orthodontics, The Royal Dental College; 1981.

[30] Riolo ML, Moyers RE, McNamara JA, Hunter WS. *An atlas of craniofacial growth: Cephalometric Standards from the University School Growth Study. Monograph No. 2, Craniofacial Growth Series, Center for Human Growth and Development.* Ann Arbor: The University of Michigan; 1974.

[31] Broadbent BH, Broadbent BH, Jr, Golden WH. *Bolton standrds of dentofacial developmental growth.* 1ª ed. Sant Louis: The C.V. Mosby Company; 1975.

[32] Bhatia SN, Leighton BC. *A manual of facial growth; a computer analysis of longitudinal cephalometric growth data.* 1ª ed. Oxford, New York: Oxford University Press; 1993.

[33] Douglas TS. *Image processing for craniofacial landmark identification and measurement: a review of photogrammetry and cephalometry.* Comput Med Imaging Graph 2004;28:401–9.

[34] Leonardi R, Giordano D, Maioran F, Spampinato C. *Automatic Cephalometric Analysis.* Angle Orthodontist 2007;78:145–51.

[35] Hermann NV, Jensen BL, Dahl E, Darvann TA, Kreiborg S. *A method for three-projection infant cephalometry.* Cleft Palate Craniofac J 2001; 38:299–316.

[36] Hermann NV, Darvann TA, Jensen BL, Dahl E, Bolund S, Kreiborg S. *Early craniofacial morphology and growth in children with bilateral complete cleft lip and palate.* Cleft Palate Craniofac Journal 2004; 41:424–38.

[37] Singh GD, Rivera-Robles Y, Jesus-Vinas J. *Longitudinal craniofacial growth patterns in patients with orofacial clefts: geometric morphometrics.* Cleft Palate Craniofac J 2004;41:136-43.

[38] Baccetti T, Franchi L, McNamara JA. *Thin-plate spline analysis of treatment effects of rapid maxillary expansion and face mask therapy in early Class III malocclusions.* Eur J Orthod 1999; 21:275-81.

[39] Halazonetis DJ. *Morphometrics for cephalometric diagnosis.* Am J Orthod Dent Orthop 2004;125:571-81.

[40] Singh GD, McNamara JA, Lozanoff S. *Thin-plate spline analysis of the cranial base in subjects with Class III malocclusion.* Eur J Orthod 1997;19:341-53.

[41] Franchi L, Baccetti T, McNamara JA. *Thin-plate spline analysis of mandibular growth.* Angle Orthod 2001;71:83-9.

[42] Houston WJB, Maher RE, McELroy D, Sherriff M. *Sources of error in measurements from cephalometric radiographs.* Eur J Orthod 1986;8:149-51.

[43] Kamoen A, Dermaut L, Verbeeck R. *The clinical significance of error measurement in the interpretation of treatment results.* Eur J Orthod 2001; 23:569-78.

[44] Maue-Dickson W. *The craniofacial complex in cleft lip and palate: an update review of anatomy and function.* Cleft Palate J 1979;16:291-317.

[45] Björk A. *Prediction of mandibular growth rotation.* Am J Orthod 1969;55:585-99.

[46] Ono I, Gunji H, Suda K, Kaneko F. *Method of preparing an exact-size model using helical volume scan computed tomography.* Plast Reconstr Surg 1994;93:1363–71.

[47] Kitaura H, Yonetsu K, Kitamori H, Kobayashi K, Nakamura T. *Standardization of 3-D CT measurements for length and angles by matrix transformation in the 3-D coordinate system.* Cleft Palate Craniofac J 2000;37:349-56.

[48] Tuncer BB, Ataç MS, Yüksel S. *A case report comparing 3-D evaluation in the diagnosis and treatment planning of hemimandibular hyperplasia with conventional radiography.* J Craniomaxillofac Surg 2009;37:312-9.

[49] Olszewski R, Cosnard G, Macq B, Mahy P, Reychler H. *Neuroradiology. 3D CT-based cephalometric analysis: 3D cephalometric theoretical concept and software.* Neuroradiology 2006;48:853-62.

[50] Terajima M, Nakasima A, Aoki Y, Goto TK, Tokumori K, Mori N, Hoshino Y. *A 3-dimensional method for analyzing the morphology of patients with maxillofacial deformities.* Am J Orthod Dentofacial Orthop 2009;136:857-67.

[51] Adams GL, Gansky SA, Miller AJ, Harrell WE Jr, Hatcher DC. *Comparison between traditional 2-dimensional cephalometry and a 3-dimensional approach on human dry skulls.* Am J Orthod Dentofacial Orthop 2004;126:397-409.

[52] Rooppakhun S, Surasith P, Vatanapatimakul N, Kaewprom Y, Sitthiseripratip K. *Craniometric study of Thai skull based on three-dimensional computed tomography (CT) data.* J Med Assoc Thai 2010;93:90-8.

[53] van Vlijmen OJ, Maal T, Bergé SJ, Bronkhorst EM, Katsaros C, Kuijpers-Jagtman AM. *A comparison between 2D and 3D cephalometry on CBCT scans of human skulls.* Int J Oral Maxillofac Surg 2010;39:156-60.

[54] Moro A, Correra P, Boniello R, Gasparini G, Pelo S. J. *Three-dimensional analysis in facial asymmetry: comparison with model analysis and conventional two-dimensional analysis.* Craniofac Surg 2009;20:417-22.

[55] Terajima M, Yanagita N, Ozeki K, Hoshino Y, Mori N, Goto TK, et al. *Three-dimensional analysis system for orthognathic surgery patients with jaw deformities.* Am J Orthod Dentofacial Orthop 2008;134:100-11.

[56] Olszewski R, Zech F, Cosnard G, Nicolas V, Macq B, Reychler H. *Three-dimensional computed tomography cephalometric craniofacial analysis: experimental validation in vitro.* Int J Oral Maxillofac Surg 2007;36:828-33.

[57] Park SH, Yu HS, Kim KD, Lee KJ, Baik HS. *A proposal for a new analysis of craniofacial morphology by 3-dimensional computed tomography.* Am J Orthod Dentofacial Orthop 2006;129:600.e23-34.

[58] Swennen GR, Schutyser F, Barth EL, De Groeve P, De Mey A. *A new method of 3-D cephalometry Part I: the anatomic Cartesian 3-D reference system.* J Craniofac Surg 2006;17:314-25.

[59] Trpkova B, Prasad NG, Lam EWN, Raboud D, Glover KE, Major PW. *Assessment of facial asymmetries from posteroanterior cephalograms: Validity of reference lines.* Am J Orthod Dentofacial Orthop 2003;123:512-20.

[60] Legrell PE, Nyquist H, Isberg A. *Validity of identification of gonion and antegonion in frontal cephalometrics.* Angle Orthod 2000;70:157-64.

[61] Habets LL, Bezuur JN, Naeiji M, Hansson TL. *The Orthopantomogram, an aid in diagnosis of temporomandibular joint problems. II. The vertical symmetry.* J Oral Rehabil 1988; 15:465-71.

194   R. M. Yáñez-Vico, D. Torres-Lagares, A. Iglesias-Linares et al.

[62] Sağlam AA, Şanli G. *Condylar Asymmetry Measurements in Patients with Temporomandibular Disorders*. J Contemp Dent Pract 2004;3:59-65.

[63] Dawson PE. *A classification system for occlusions that relates maximal intercuspation to the position and condition of the temporomandibular joints.* J Prosthet Dent 1996;75: 60–6.

[64] Van Elslande DC, Russett SJ , Major PW, Flores-Mird C. *Mandibular asymmetry diagnosis with panoramic imaging.* Am J Orthod Dentofacial Orthop 2008;134:183-92.

[65] Williamson PC, Mayor PW, Nebbe B, Glover KE, West K. *Landmark identification error in submentovertex cephalometrics.* Oral Surg Oral Med Oral Pathol Oral Radiol Endod 1998;86:360-9.

[66] Lysell L, Petersson A. *The submento-vertex projection in radiography of the temporomandibular joint.* Dentomaxillofac Radiol 1980; 9: 11-7.

[67] Park W, Kim BC, Yu HS, Yi CK, Lee SH. *Architectural characteristics of the normal and deformity mandible revealed by three-dimensional functional unit analysis.* Clin Oral Investig 2010;14:691-8.

[68] Hwang HS, Hwang CH, Lee KH, Kang BC. *Maxillofacial 3-dimensional image analysis for the diagnosis of facial asymmetry.* Am J Orthod Dentofacial Orthop 2006;130:779-85.

[69] Michiels G, Sather AH. *Determinants of facial attractiveness in a sample of white women.* Int J Adult Orthodon Orthgnath Surg 1994:9:95-103.

[70] Cho BC, Shin DP, Park JW, Baik BS. *Bimaxillary osteodistraction for the treatment of facial asymmetry in adults.* Br J Plast Surg 2001;54:491-8.

[71] Rachmiel A, Manor R, Peled M, Laufer D. *Intraoral distraction osteogenesis of the mandible in hemifacial microsoma.* J Oral Maxillofac Surg 2001;59:728-33.

[72] Marsh]L, Vannier MW. *Three-dimensional surface imaging from CT scans for the study of craniofacial dysmorphology (review).* I Craniofac Genet Dev Biol 1989;9:61-75.

[73] Altobelli DE, Kikinis R, Mulliken IB, Cline H, Lorensen WF, lolesz F. *Computer-assisted three-dimensional planning in craniofacial surgery.* Plast Reconstr Surg 1993;92:576-85.

[74] Posnick JC, Goldstein JA, Waitzman AA. *Surgical correction of the Treacher Collins malar deficiency: quantitative CT scan analysis of long-term results.* Plast Reconstr Surg 1993;92:12-22.

3D-CT in Oral and Maxillofacial Research 195

[75] Olszewski R, Zech F, Cosnard G, Nicolas V, Macq B, Reychler H. *Three-dimensional computed tomography cephalometric craniofacial analysis: experimental validation in vitro.* Int J Oral Maxillofac Surg 2007;36:828-33.

[76] Kitaura H, Yonetsu K, Kitamori H, Kobayashi K, Nakamura T. *Standardization of 3-D CT measurements for length and angles by matrix transformation in the 3-D coordinate system.* Cleft Palate Craniofac J 2000;37:349-56.

[77] Glat PM, Freund RM, Spector JA, Levine J, Noz M, Bookstein FL, et al. *A classification of plagiocephaly utilizing a three-dimensional computer analysis of cranial base landmarks.* Ann Plast Surg 1996;36:469–74.

[78] Shortliffe E, Perreault LE, Wiederhold G, Fagan LM. *Medical informatics: computer applications in health care and biomedicine.* 2nd ed. New York: Springer; 2001.

[79] Kapila S, Conley RS, Harrell WE Jr. *The current status of cone beam computed tomography imaging in orthodontics.* Dentomaxillofac Radiol 2011;40:24-34.

In: CT Scans
Editors: V. E. Perkel et al.

ISBN 978-1-62100-319-9
©2011 Nova Science Publishers, Inc.

Chapter 6

OVERDENTURE CONSTRUCTION OF IMPLANTS DIRECTIONALLY PLACED USING CT SCANNING TECHNIQUES

Timothy F. Kosinski[*]
University of Detroit Mercy School of Dentistry, Detroit, MI, U. S.

ABSTRACT

CT scanning software is fast becoming a viable tool in the diagnosing of dental implant position and placement. Minimally invasive procedures may be requested by patients to reduce their anxiety and increase treatment acceptance rates. In areas where contours and width and height of bone are difficult to determine with conventional radiographic techniques, the CT scanning software allows diagnostic determination if bone quantity and quality exists and can be used to virtually place dental implants using the computer program prior to any surgical intervention. This is an outstanding tool in discussing the risks involved in surgical implant procedures and can help visualize the case finished before ever starting. Used in critical anatomic situations and for placing the implant in an ideal position in bone, CT scanning software eliminates possible manual placement errors and matches planning to prosthetic requirements. This innovative tool makes surgical placement of implants less invasive and more predictable. Prosthetic reconstruction is

---

[*] Correspondence Author: Timothy Kosinski 248 545-8651 or drkosin@aol.com 31000 Telegraph Rd., Ste. 170 Bingham Farms, MI 48025

thus made simpler since the implants are appropriately positioned to allow for fabrication of the final prosthesis.

Keywords: Easyguide, Straumann Implant, Bredent attachment

Fabrication of a stable, comfortable maxillary removable complete denture using dental implants as the support mechanism begins with careful diagnosis and case planning. Simple two dimensional images created using conventional radiographic techniques may no longer be an adequate and predictable technique for proper implant placement. The surgeon's experience and manual placement techniques greatly influences the final functional and esthetic result. Any laboratory technician can tell you that often implants are placed in poor position or angulation making prosthetic fabrication difficult or retention comprosised.

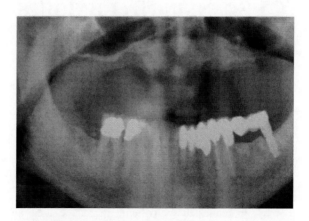

Figure 1.

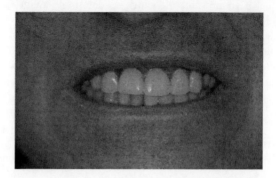

Figure 2.

Dental implants provide an outstanding treatment option demonstrating dramatic improvement in denture stability and increased chewing efficiency. There is an increase in quality of life that is rewarding to the dentist and gratifying for the patient. The use of endosseous implant designs, such as the Straumann dental implant system, has proven to have an outstanding prognosis and are reliable as retainers for overdentures.

This patient is a 68 year old white male who has worn a conventional maxillary complete denture opposing natural and implant retained dentition for many years. There are no medical contraindications to dental implant therapy. Following maxillary tooth removal several maxillary complete dentures were fabricated over the years which were not completely acceptable to the patient both functionally and esthetically. Form and function diminished over the years and the patient was anxious for a stable maxillary dentition.

Several options were discussed with the patient including fabrication of another new conventional case. The posterior vertical bone was minimal due to the large maxillary sinuses. The amount of anterior pre-maxillary bone was difficult to determine by radiographic interpretation alone. The patient's main concern was that the existing maxillary case was not stable and his ability to chew and function had diminished. His quality of life had been compromised by the loss of his upper teeth. Discussion of the use of CT technology to determine the exact amount of bone available and the use of CT scanning software to determine precise position of potential implants helped motivate the patient to consider dental implant reconstruction.

There was significant facial resorption in the maxilla, so it was determined that an implant retained maxillary overdenture with proper lip support would best serve the patient. Struamann Dental Implants (Struamann Corp,, Boston) were chosen due to their long term successes. This system improves the dentist's and patient's access to superior and more effective treatment. Reliability and innovation are two strong qualities of the Straumann surgical and prosthetic techniques that made this the implant of choice in this situation. The implant provides an 8 degree Morse taper internal connection. The flared neck implant design used here is ideal for soft tissue contouring.

There are often concerns with any surgical procedures, especially in the sinus area or in bone where nerves are located. These concerns have popularized a newer concept in implant dentistry. We are now able to utilize our CAD/CAM computer software to visualize the patient's entire mouth anatomy in three dimensions, which takes all of ten minutes. The computer software allows us to simulate the placement of implants accurately before ever touching the patient. A surgical guide, created from the three dimensional images, helps us place the dental implants in the proper pre-determined positions, often without ever making a flap incision. This technique is proving to be a cost effective solution to assist the implant dentist in planning an esthetic and functional final result and minimizing any surgical challenges they may face.

The CAD/CAM technology is based on planning algorithms used clinically for more than 11 years. CT scans and 3D planning software can really improve our predictability and safety. The CAD/CAM techniques can be used for single tooth edentulous spaces, single tooth immediate extraction cases, partially edentulous spaces, fully edentulous maxillary and mandibular overdenture cases or fully edentulous maxillary or mandibular full arch permanent restorations. The surgical cases are, therefore, driven by the final esthetic and functional result. It is important to listen to your patients carefully to determine their goals and desires and design the implant reconstruction accordingly. It is critical today to make sure that the final tooth reconstruction is established before any surgical intervention. Placing the dental implants in the jaw before understanding tooth/implant position and the final result is a big mistake. [1,3,4]

The CAD/CAM planning and placement system provides a high level of comfort and safety for the patient by reducing surgical and restorative time. This is done by utilizing an accurate three dimensional plan prior to implant placement. There are obvious advantages including; easy visual understanding for clear case presentations, reduced surgical chair time, reduced restorative chair time in certain cases because of ideal implant positioning, reduced stress for the clinician and the patient, the avoidance of surprises during surgery, optimal implant placement for long term implant and prosthetic success and , most importantly, an improved esthetic result.

Prior to the CT scan a radiographic guide is fabricated by the dentist, which aids in visualization of the optimal prosthetic outcome. The teeth are positioned properly in wax and then a hard model to illustrate what the case will look like finished before ever starting. All appropriate dental anatomy is included. The radiographic guide is placed in the mouth during the CT scan. This allows the clinician to see the ideal position of the teeth on a three dimensional model. The entire 3D image is analyzed and the implant planning and simulation of implant placement completed using the computer. The surgical placement of the implants can be done in a conventional manner using the newly created surgical guide to help direct the implants in the ideal position, but surgery can often be completed without making any incisional flap. The implants are placed in the desired depth using the computer software and the surgical guide.

It is imperative that the implants be placed as nearly parallel in all three dimensions, as possible, to the long axis of the bone and to each other. The implants in the right maxilla are parallel to each other as are the implants in the left maxilla. Due to the arch form it may be difficult to parallel all six implants sequentially. A clear surgical stent was fabricated using the information created using the CT scanning software. The guide is used to correctly position the implants in the first molar and cuspid areas to maximize stability of the final implant retained prosthesis No retraction of the soft tissue was needed, since the CT indicated in three dimensions the length and width and position of the implants to be used..

Figures 1 illustrates the loss of posterior maxillary bone and irregular shaped pattern of the pre maxillary bone making implant placement difficult to determine. Without CT diagnosis it may be speculated that adequate bone height and width exists, but this could not be exactly determined until a complete periodontal flap is made and surgical placement would be dictated by the experience of the implant dentist. Figure 2 illustrates the existing conventional maxillary complete denture with a closed vertical dimension of occlusion resulting in improper lip support and a poor frontal and lateral esthetic profile. The patients decrease in function may be due to the poor plane of occlusion and tooth position. Gagging was caused by the basic design of the conventional denture and poor fit. Quality of life was dramatically reduced. Figures 3 and 4 show how the CT scanning software is used to virtually place six anterior implants , their angulation and how the implants will be restored. In properly virtually placing the implants it was noted that the right and left arches would not allow parallelism of all six implants, so the three right side implants would be splinted together and the left side implants would be splinted separately. To achieve the best functional and esthetic result, as well as increase stability of any prosthesis, it was decided to parallel the implants as possible and place them in the pre-maxillary area and as posterior as the bone would allow. This is all determined virtually prior to any surgical intervention, a tremendous advantage to the less experienced implant surgeon.

Prior to the preparation of the osteotomies, the surgical directional guide is created with guiding openings in the stent. (Figure 5)This allows the pilot drill to penetrate the stent, through the soft tissue into the bone to a predetermined depth. Once the pilot drill makes an mark into the soft tissue and bone, a flap was made to visualize the precise contours of bone. The remaining osteotomies into the bone are made for the six implants chosen. The drills are used at approximately 800 RPM to the hub of the bur. 4.1mm X 10mm Straumann implants are threaded to place following the contours of the arch. (Figures 6,7) A radiograph is made of the implants in position (Figure 8) Remember depth into bone has been determined by the CT scanning softwsare. All angles are also predetermined with the virtual placement of the implants.

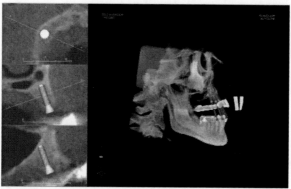

Figure 3.

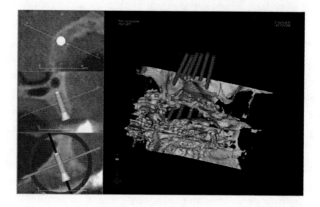

Figure 4.

Overdenture Construction of Implants Directionally Placed ... 203

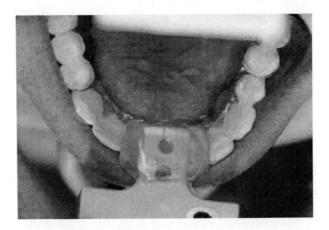

Figure 5.

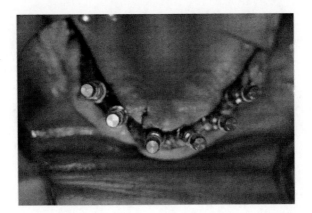

Figure 6.

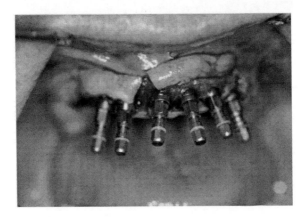

Figure 7.

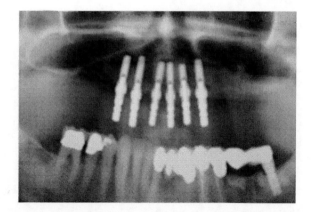

Figure 8.

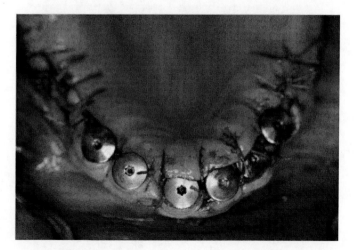

Figure 9.

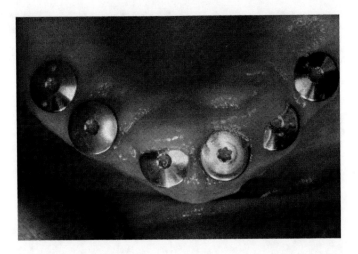

Figure 10.

The shoulder of the implants are left slightly coronal to the crestal bone to allow for easy access. 1.5mm tall closure screws were placed into each implant. (Figure 9) and the flap sutured closed using Vicryl sutures. Following three months of integration the tissue around the closure screws are pink and firm. (Figure 10) A closed custom tray impression of the implants was made using the Straumann impression cap and synOcta positioning cylinders.(Figure 11) A master impression was sent to the lab to have the proper analogs placed into the impression and placed into the impression for a master model pour up. The master cast is poured duplicating all peripheral borders. A bite registration was used to position the casts. Teeth are positioned to esthetics and function.

The Bredent (XPdent Corp.) attachments are intended to act as retentive devices for this overdenture case. Because of their design and incorporation into two screw retained bars the patient is able to easily align and seat the overdentures easily. Although not critical in bar fabrication, it is better that the implants be placed in a nearly parallel position to each other, to simplify the prosthetic construction. According to the manufacturer, the attachments are the most flexible and simplest attachment system on the market. There are three levels of retention to meet the needs of any individual and eventual changing of the attachments following wear is easily accomplished. [2]

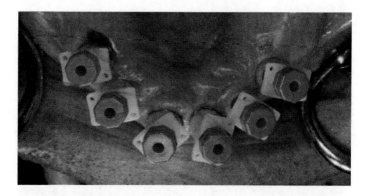

Figure 11.

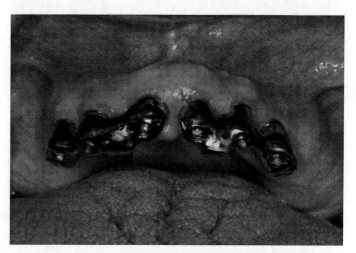

Figure 12.

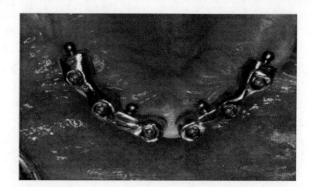

Figure 13.

When selecting an appropriate attachment for the overdenture, it is important to consider the amount of interocclusal space available. Retention requirements, ease of use and lifespan of attachment are also considered. One of the main benefits of the Bredent attachment is their reliability of retention and ease of use. The retentive mechanism is based on plastic female components that sit in a metal housing. The attachments come in three retentions, green is the least retentive, yellow next and red the most retentive. Since four attachments were used in this case, yellow was chosen as retentive enough.

Conventional denture techniques are used to create the final esthetic contours. We create an outstanding functional and esthetic result, meet the patient's expectations and totally eliminate the gagging reflex caused by the old full palate conventional complete denture.

Figures 12 and 13 illustrate the facial and coronal position of the two screw retained bars, separated at the midline. Figure 14 is a close up of the male portion of the Bredent attachment. Figures 15 and 16 show the yellow attachment in metal housing in the palateless (horseshoe shaped) maxillary prosthesis. The shape of the denture completely eliminates any gagging reflex and tremendously imporoves taste sensation. A final panoramic radiograph (figure 16) shows the bars in place. Fortunately there was plenty of room for a bar design. If interocclusal clearance was a problem, a different attachment, such as the Locator type, would have been considered. Connecting the maxillary implants with bars improves the support and stablility of the implants placed in the relatively soft maxillary bone. It is this author's opinion that splinting the implants in the maxillary improves the long term prognosis of the implants themselves. Figure 17 is the final radiograph with the two bars in place. Note the smooth transition from metal framework to implant body.

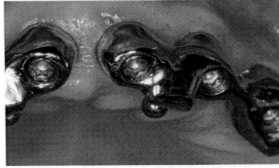

Figure 14.

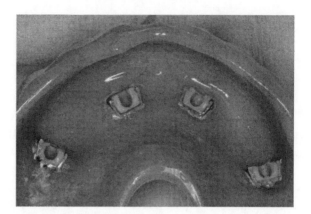

Figure 15.

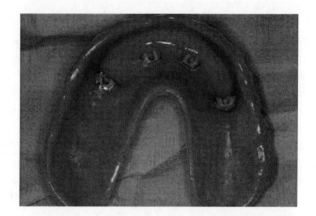

Figure 16.

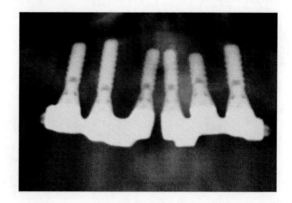

Figure 17.

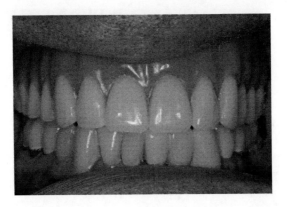

Figure 18.

This type of prosthesis allows for excellent retention and stability for this patient. The Bredent attachments are positioned extracoronally on two bars separated at the midline. This allows for good palatal tissue adaptation and easy maintenance with a simple tooth brush or end-tuft brush. Follow up care includes clinical assessment for abutment stability, mobility of the implants and plaque accumulation. Since the perimucosal seal is vital to protect the underlying connective tissue and borne from migrating forces, probing a healthy implant is not advised. Radiographs are taken yearly to determine bone position and contour. Metal scalers and ultrasonic instruments may scar and pit the titanium abutment surface, therefore, plastic, gold or graphite scalers should be used as necessary.

This patient exhibited a positive end result because of his understanding of the limiting factors involved in this case and the final prosthesis. He is, however, able to chew more efficiently and speak clearly without worry of the prosthesis loosening or any of the abutments decaying. Quality of life was dramatically improved using an implant retained overdenture. .Figures 18, 19,20 and 21 illustrate the final esthetic results.

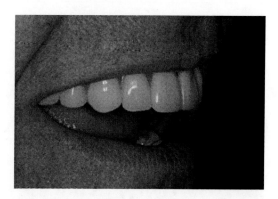

Figure 19.

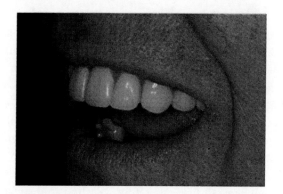

Figure 20.

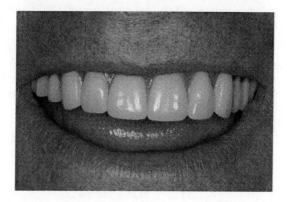

Figure 21.

The general dentist has an obligation to provide his/her patients with the most innovative, proven techniques available. CT scans and scanning software

Overdenture Construction of Implants Directionally Placed ... 211

like the Keystone Easyguide program makes surgical placement of the dental implants rather routine. Anatomical anomalies are virtually determined prior to ever touching the patient. With better implant placement comes more routine and predictable prosthetic reconstruction. Since the GP is the professional the patient consults concerning their dental condition, he/she must educate himself with the treatment modalities. Many surgical therapies can be performed by the trained general dentist and certainly all general dentists should be able to restore these cases simply and easily. The predictable results only reinforces the modality. Maintenance is rather routine with a design of the bars that allows easy access with a proxy brush. As with any other dental appliance, professional evaluations and periodic radiographs are mandated.

ACKNOWLEDGEMENT

Dr. Kosinski is an Adjunct Assistant Professor at the University of Detroit Mercy School of Dentistry and serves on the editorial review board of *Reality*, the information source for esthetic dentistry, Contemporary Esthetics and Clinical Advisors, and became the editor of the Michigan Academy of General Dentistry. Dr. Kosinski received his DDS from the University of Detroit Mercy Dental School and his Mastership in Biochemistry from Wayne State University School of Medicine. He is a Diplomat of the American Board of Oral Implantology/Implant Dentistry, the International Congress of Oral Implantologists and the American Society of Osseointegration. He is a Fellow of the American Academy of Implant Dentistry and received his Mastership in the Academy of General Dentistry. Dr. Kosinski has received many honors including Fellowship in the American and International Colleges of Dentists and the Academy of Dentistry International. He is a member of OKU and the Pierre Fauchard Academy. Dr. Kosinski was the University of Detroit Mercy School of Dentistry Alumni Association's "Alumnus of the Year." Dr. Kosinski has published over 55 articles on the surgical and prosthetic phases of implant dentistry and was a contributor to the textbook, Principles and Practices of Implant Dentistry.

REFERENCES

Int. J of Oral and Maxillofacial Implants. Vol. 18. No. 6, 2003. *Image Guided Systems Provided a Reliable Preoperative Assessment of Implant Size and Anatomic Complications.*

JCDA. Vol. 73, No. 8, 2007 *Point of Care: How Do I Select An Attachment for use in a Removable Partial Denture or Overdenture.*

Clinical Oral Implants Res. Vol. 13, 2002. *Precision of Transfer of Preoperative Planning for Oral Implants Based on Cone Beam CT Scan Images Through a Robotic Drilling Machine: An In Vitro Study.*

Int. J. Oral and Maxillofacial Implants. Vol. 21, No. 2, 2006. *Minimally Invasive Procedures May Be Requested By Patients to Reduce Anxiety and the Pain Experienced.*

INDEX

A

access, 26, 46, 179, 199, 205, 211
acetic acid, 57
acid, 114, 152
acoustic neuroma, 137, 146
acoustics, 137
acquaintance, 135
acquisitions, 175
acute renal failure, 68
adaptation, 209
adenosine, 96, 107
adjustment, 44, 46
adults, 96, 107, 108, 194
advancement, ix, 24, 26, 34, 44, 47, 174
age, 100, 121, 123, 134, 145
algorithm, 37, 78, 80, 170
allergy, 29, 83
amalgam, 176
American Heart Association, 104, 108
anastomosis, 19, 91
anatomy, 93, 94, 95, 96, 100, 106, 107, 135, 154, 155, 159, 179, 180, 192, 199, 200
anemia, 140
aneurysm, 27, 111, 114, 115, 116, 121, 122, 124, 143, 144, 148, 151, 152, 153, 155, 156, 157, 158, 159, 160
angina, 83
angiogram, 86, 89, 115, 131, 132, 153, 158
angiography, viii, 70, 73, 79, 82, 83, 84, 86, 87, 88, 89, 91, 92, 96, 101, 102, 103, 104, 105, 106, 108, 115, 132, 143, 144, 148, 150, 154, 155, 157, 158, 159, 160, 161, 171
angulation, 183, 198, 201
anisocytosis, 113, 151
anxiety, x, 38, 197
aorta, 28, 82, 92, 94, 96
apnea, 129
appendicitis, viii, ix, 109, 112, 147, 150
arteries, 28, 133, 158, 159, 161, 162, 163, 165, 168
arteriogram, 92
arterioles, 114, 152
arteriovenous malformation, 128, 130, 132
artery, 82, 83, 84, 86, 87, 88, 89, 90, 91, 92, 96, 100, 102, 103, 104, 105, 111, 114, 115, 120, 121, 122, 125, 133, 144, 148, 150, 151, 152, 153, 155, 156, 158, 160, 161, 162, 163, 165, 168, 172
ascites, 19, 24, 64, 66
assessment, 25, 26, 52, 67, 68, 73, 74, 77, 84, 86, 95, 96, 99, 102, 104, 105, 165, 166, 186, 188
asymmetry, 179, 184, 186, 189, 190, 194
asymptomatic, 88, 100, 125
atherosclerosis, 105, 134
atherosclerotic plaque, 88, 100, 105
atrial fibrillation, 82, 83, 94, 106, 107
atrium, 93, 94
attachment, 198, 205, 207
Austria, 1
autopsy, 133
avoidance, 200

Index

B

background radiation, 97
backscattering, 25
bacteria, 22
ban, 161
base, 34, 69, 75, 168, 179, 184, 187, 192, 195
basilar artery, 162, 165, 168
bending, 48
benefits, 100, 122, 141, 148, 180, 184, 207
benign, 50, 133, 146
beta blocker, 82
bile, 2, 7, 19, 22, 64
bile duct, 2, 7, 19, 22, 64
biochemistry, 129
biomarkers, 90
biopsy, 71, 74, 75, 76, 77
bleeding, 2, 23, 115, 118, 119, 124, 135, 142, 153
bone, x, 114, 152, 170, 177, 181, 183, 184, 187, 197, 199, 201, 205, 207, 209
bone marrow, 114, 152
bones, viii, ix, 109, 112, 147, 149, 173, 177, 179, 185
bowel, 22
brain, ix, 75, 76, 115, 133, 135, 136, 140, 147, 152, 153, 172
brain stem, 133, 135
brainstem, 145
breast cancer, 3, 56
breathing, 29, 37
bronchospasm, 82
bundle branch block, 102
burn, 97, 113, 151

C

cadaver, 72
calcification, 83, 86, 88, 103, 154, 155, 159, 160
calcifications, 84
calcium, viii, 79, 82, 83, 84, 88, 105
calcium channel blocker, 82
caliber, 83, 90, 91
calibration, 48
canals, 187
cancer, 63, 97, 108, 119
candidates, 56, 180, 187
capillary, 138
capsule, 7, 15, 22, 23, 24
carcinogenesis, 97
carcinoma, 3, 51, 59, 66, 77
cardiac arrhythmia, 94
cardiac catheterization, 123
cardiovascular disease, viii, ix, 96, 109, 112, 147, 150
cardiovascular risk, 105
caricature, 170
catheter, 37, 64, 84, 93, 94, 106, 107, 113, 119, 151, 154, 155, 159
cerebellum, 133
cerebral aneurysm, 128, 130, 155
cerebral arteries, 114, 144, 151
cerebral blood flow, 142
cerebral contusion, 140
cerebral hemisphere, 114, 134, 152
cerebrospinal fluid, 113, 151
cerebrovascular disease, 144
challenges, 55, 70, 76, 200
channel blocker, 82
charring, 9
chemotherapy, 54, 78
childhood, 146
children, 96, 140, 146, 181, 187, 191
China, 68, 141
cholangiocarcinoma, 56
chromosome, 133
chronic renal failure, 26
circulation, 116, 121, 153, 166, 167, 172
cirrhosis, 24, 57, 70
clarity, viii, ix, 109, 112, 147, 149
classification, 89, 119, 120, 123, 194, 195
cleft lip, 181, 186, 191, 192
closure, 205
clusters, 16
coagulopathy, 119, 140
coarctation, 96
cocaine, 122, 123, 124, 144
cochlear implant, 41

Index

cognitive abilities, 135
collaboration, 128, 130
collagen, 140
collateral, vii, 1, 20, 22, 38, 41, 49, 134, 164
collateral damage, vii, 1, 38, 41
colon, 22
color, 24, 87, 176
colorectal cancer, 3, 55, 56, 58, 68
coma, 133
communication, 175
compensation, 38, 73, 75, 189
complement, 96, 155, 159
complexity, 167
compliance, 124
complications, vii, 1, 2, 20, 36, 38, 39, 48, 49, 50, 55, 57, 63, 64, 94, 131, 132, 144, 158
compression, 133, 145
computed tomography, vii, ix, 1, 71, 77, 85, 86, 88, 89, 91, 93, 94, 95, 101, 102, 103, 104, 105, 106, 107, 108, 150, 155, 169, 173, 174, 175, 181, 185, 187, 189, 190, 192, 193, 195
computer, viii, ix, x, 35, 46, 64, 70, 74, 101, 107, 109, 112, 147, 149, 179, 180, 190, 191, 195, 197, 199, 200
computer software, 199, 201
computing, 41, 70
conduction, 3
conductivity, 4
configuration, 26
congenital heart disease, 96, 107, 108
connective tissue, 209
conscious sedation, 20
consensus, 18, 105, 166
construction, vii, 205
consumption, 118, 142
contour, 209
contradiction, 162
control group, 25, 128, 130, 180
controversial, 95, 100
controversies, 70
cooling, 5, 9, 14, 18, 22, 23, 59, 64
cooperation, 38, 161
coordination, 44
correlation, 25, 27, 66, 67, 123, 137

correlation coefficient, 25
cortex, 133
cost, 90, 183, 184, 200
covering, 39, 137, 175
cranial nerve, 120, 135, 137
craniotomy, 120
critical analysis, 146, 171
cytology, 36
cytoplasm, 138

D

danger, 7, 38, 124
data analysis, 128, 130
data set, 81, 82, 88, 92, 96, 130
data transfer, 42, 46, 48
deaths, 140
defects, 95
deficiency, 187, 194
deficit, 120
deformation, 27, 38
degradation, 113, 151
denaturation, 50
dental implants, x, 74, 197, 198, 200, 211
dentist, 199, 200, 201, 210
dentures, 199
deposition, 3, 9, 16, 114, 115, 116, 152, 153
depth, 29, 44, 45, 76, 201
destruction, 135
detectable, 26, 117
detection, 26, 27, 51, 54, 66, 67, 84, 85, 86, 87, 88, 90, 102, 103, 104
deviation, 41, 43, 179, 185, 186
diaphragm, 22, 60, 66
diastole, 97
differential diagnosis, 116, 133
diffusion, 5, 14, 15, 17, 22, 23
diseases, viii, ix, 110, 112, 115, 128, 129, 130, 147, 150, 153
disorder, 116, 133
disseminated intravascular coagulation, 115, 117, 140, 153
distortions, 47, 74
distribution, 15
dizziness, 116, 133, 153

Index

drainage, 71, 106
drawing, ix, 173
drug abuse, 144

E

ecchymosis, 113, 114, 117, 119, 151, 152, 154
electrical conductivity, 14, 61
electrocautery, 60
electrode surface, 3, 6, 7
electrodes, 5, 6, 7, 8, 9, 10, 12, 14, 15, 16, 17, 18, 21, 22, 23, 24, 37, 41, 48, 49, 57, 60, 61, 62, 63, 76
electromagnetic, 34, 36, 37, 40, 41, 44, 47, 73, 74, 75
electron, 81
electrons, 81
emboli, 134
embolism, 134
embolus, 133
emergency, 125
emission, 86, 104
endoscopy, 65, 69
endothelial cells, 115, 152, 153
energy, 3, 9, 15, 16, 17, 37, 55, 65, 81
enforcement, 27
engineering, 69, 70
entropy, 29
environment, 40, 69, 125
epidural hematoma, 118
epilepsy, 76
epithelium, 138
equilibrium, 25
equipment, viii, ix, 27, 109, 112, 147, 149
error management, 74
esophagus, 94, 107
ethanol, 56, 57, 59, 69
evidence, 96, 100, 114, 116, 125, 131, 138, 152, 168
examinations, 162
excision, 138
exclusion, 65
exercise, 87
exposure, 49, 54, 58, 71, 81, 89, 96, 97, 98, 99, 108, 155, 184

external magnetic fields, 41
extraction, 200

F

fabrication, x, 198, 199, 205
Fabrication, 198
facial asymmetry, 185, 186, 189, 193, 194
faith, 184
false negative, 54, 132, 137, 158
false positive, 158
families, 137
fat, 163
fear, 100
fever, 2
fibrillation, 82, 106
fibrin, 113, 114, 116, 151, 152, 153
fibrinogen, 113, 118, 151
fibrinolysis, 115, 153
fibrinolytic, 112, 115, 116, 143, 150, 152, 153
fibrosis, 26, 69
fibrous tissue, 5
filament, 139
films, 179
filters, 150
filtration, 26
first molar, 186, 201
fistulas, 22
fixation, 34, 37, 38, 76
flight, 148, 149, 161
flights, 41
fluid, 113, 151
foramen, 75, 76
foramen ovale, 75, 76
Ford, 77
formation, 18, 22, 115, 124, 153
fragments, 27
freedom, 44, 46
freezing, 81
functional changes, 77, 145
functional imaging, 54, 100
fusion, 7, 28, 29, 41, 48, 49, 50, 70, 71

Index

G

gadolinium, 26
gallbladder, 22, 64
gastrointestinal tract, 64
gel, 48
general anaesthesia, 20
general anesthesia, 20, 38
genotype, 137
geometry, x, 59, 60, 174, 178
Germany, 45, 119
glucose, 22, 54, 78
grading, 123, 124
granules, 115, 152, 153
graphite, 209
grounding, 15, 16, 58
growth, 5, 180, 181, 187, 190, 191, 192
guidance, vii, 1, 2, 24, 25, 26, 28, 29, 30, 31,
    32, 34, 40, 41, 43, 44, 45, 55, 60, 69, 71,
    72, 74, 75
guidelines, 20, 63

H

hard tissues, 188
head injury, 118, 140, 143
head trauma, 118, 119
headache, 113, 116, 120, 121, 150, 153
health, vii, 97, 99, 146, 195
health care, 195
health risks, vii, 99
heart disease, 96, 100, 103
heart rate, 80, 81, 82, 84, 90, 97, 102, 104
height, x, 185, 186, 197, 201
hematoma, 114, 116, 118, 135, 143, 152
hemiparesis, 113, 116, 120, 151, 154
hemisphere, 34
hemorrhage, 20, 113, 114, 118, 120, 123, 140,
    143, 151, 152, 159
hemorrhagic stroke, 135, 146
hemostasis, 115, 142, 153
hepatocellular carcinoma, 2, 56, 57, 59, 60,
    63, 64, 66, 67, 68, 69, 70, 72, 77
hernia, 22

histological examination, 138
history, 104, 113, 144, 150
housing, 207
hub, 202
human, 47, 144, 163, 176, 190, 193
human body, 163
Hunter, 191
hybrid, 72, 87, 104
hyperemia, 50
hyperplasia, 68, 192
hypertonic saline, 61, 62
hypofibrinogenemia, 118
hypotension, 82
hypothesis, 112

I

iatrogenic, 22
ideal, x, 184, 185, 197, 199, 200
identification, 27, 94, 174, 176, 177, 184, 185,
    188, 190, 191, 193, 194
idiopathic, 169
imaging modalities, 54, 95, 98, 100, 162
immobilization, viii, 2, 73
immunity, 142
implant placement, 198, 200, 201, 211
implant planning, 200
implants, vii, x, 27, 197, 198, 199, 200, 201,
    205, 207, 209
in vitro, 5, 61, 75, 77, 190, 193, 195
in vivo, 59, 60, 62, 63, 69, 76, 77
incidence, 137, 138
individuals, 88, 89, 98, 103
infarction, 133, 134, 145
infection, 19, 22, 47, 50
infundibulum, 155, 160
injuries, viii, ix, 64, 109, 112, 140, 147, 150
injury, 2, 15, 22, 60, 64, 70, 117, 118, 135,
    140, 146
insertion, 25, 36, 47, 48, 93
integration, 54, 70, 94, 205
intensity values, 35
interface, 40, 52
interference, 40
interpersonal contact, 135

intervention, 2, 27, 34, 37, 39, 44, 45, 46, 71, 124, 130, 131, 132, 143, 159
intestinal perforation, 2
intestine, 20
intracranial aneurysm, 112, 124, 143, 144, 145, 155, 157, 158, 160, 171
inversion, 66
iodine, 82
ionizing radiation, 24, 26, 97, 98
ions, 3
iron, 70
ischemia, 50, 83, 87, 115, 116, 153, 168
issues, 48, 97, 135
Italy, 141, 142, 171

J

Japan, 57
joints, 44, 45, 194

L

laboratory studies, 117
laceration, 38
laparoscopy, 22
latency, 97
lead, 7, 18, 22, 23, 25, 38, 86, 95, 177, 181
left atrium, 93, 94, 106, 107
legs, 117, 154
lesions, vii, 1, 5, 7, 9, 14, 21, 22, 23, 24, 25, 26, 28, 34, 35, 36, 43, 52, 54, 59, 67, 68, 71, 73, 87, 89, 90, 92, 100, 102, 104, 105, 118, 132, 133
lifetime, 98
light, 40, 113, 151, 186
local anesthetic, 122
localization, 25, 29, 47, 87, 184, 189
loci, 118
longevity, 100
low risk, 2
lumen, 83, 88, 91, 114, 152
lutetium, 78
lying, 113, 151
lysis, 113, 151

M

magnetization, 163
majority, 177, 178, 181
malignancy, 55, 97, 98
malignant tumors, 137
malocclusion, 181, 192
man, 86, 100, 115, 121, 153
management, 26, 56, 58, 72, 76, 117, 119, 124, 125, 128, 130, 154
mandible, 181, 185, 187, 190, 194
manipulation, ix, 29, 173
mapping, 94, 106
mass, 98, 133, 138
master model, 205
mastoid, 184
matrix, 176, 192, 195
matter, iv, 92, 164, 168
maxilla, 181, 187, 199, 201
maxillary sinus, 199
media, 29, 68, 83
medical, vii, viii, ix, 2, 41, 73, 79, 97, 109, 110, 112, 117, 125, 130, 145, 147, 148, 149, 154, 167, 199
medical robots, viii, 2
medicine, 74, 97, 103, 104, 119, 129
medulla, 133
medulla oblongata, 133
messenger RNA, 137
meta-analysis, 66
metabolites, 144
metastasis, 78
mice, 66
microcirculation, 25
midbrain, 111, 135, 136, 148
migraine headache, 137
miniature, 47
models, 21, 41, 164, 174, 185, 187, 188
modifications, 165
molecular biology, 137
morbidity, 2, 22, 54, 120, 140
morphology, 180, 191, 192, 193
mortality, 2, 54, 55, 118, 120, 121, 140, 145
mortality rate, 2, 54, 121
motion control, viii, 2, 38, 39, 72

Index

mucous membrane, 114, 152
multiple factors, 81
mutations, 137
myocardial infarction, 95, 107, 122
myocardial ischemia, 92
myocyte, 107

N

nasogastric tube, 117
nausea, 133
navigation system, vii, 2, 35, 39, 40, 41, 42, 43, 44, 46, 48, 69, 73, 74, 75
necrosis, viii, 2, 3, 5, 6, 9, 14, 15, 16, 17, 18, 21, 23, 24, 49, 51, 52, 53, 54, 59, 62, 65
negative effects, 23
nephropathy, 83
nerve, 120, 137
nervous system, 142
neuroma, 137
neurons, 129
neuroscience, 129
neurosurgery, 39, 72, 128, 130, 145, 160
neutrophils, 113, 151
nitrates, 82
nitrogen, 113, 151
nodules, 24
noncalcified, 88, 89
nuchal rigidity, 113, 120, 151
nystagmus, 133

O

obesity, 54
obstacles, 18, 19, 20, 41
obstruction, 89, 96, 107
occlusion, 131, 133, 145, 150, 155, 156, 157, 161, 162, 164, 165, 166, 167, 168, 171, 201
occult blood, 117, 154
old age, 119
opacification, 165, 166, 168
opportunities, 55
optical systems, 41
organ, 18, 22, 29, 37, 42

organize, 124
organs, vii, viii, ix, 15, 22, 29, 79, 109, 112, 147, 149
orthodontic treatment, 183
osteotomy, 190
ostium, 93
overweight, 78
oxygen, 20, 123

P

pain, 7, 20, 22, 38, 50, 84, 86, 90, 100, 105, 113, 122, 150
palate, 181, 186, 191, 192, 207
papilledema, 113, 151
parallel, viii, 18, 20, 35, 79, 161, 177, 201, 205
parallelism, 201
parenchyma, 15, 24
paresis, 140
partial thromboplastin time, 113, 151
participants, 125
pathology, 74, 133, 159
pathophysiology, 135
perforation, 22, 23, 50
perfusion, 5, 14, 15, 18, 22, 27, 59, 60, 86, 87, 95, 96, 100, 104, 107, 134
pericardium, 114, 152
periodontal, 201
peripheral blood, 113, 151
peritoneal cavity, 114, 152
peritoneum, 22
permeation, 138
permission, 80, 85, 86, 87, 88, 89, 91, 92, 93, 94, 95, 98, 99, 141
petechiae, 117, 154
phenotype, 137
phenotypes, 137
photons, x, 174, 177
physicians, viii, ix, 16, 109, 112, 133, 147, 149
physics, 72, 73, 74, 101
physiological factors, 95
pigs, 16
pilot study, 62, 76

Index

pitch, 81, 170
plaque, 88, 89, 90, 105, 209
plasminogen, 115, 116, 149, 152, 153
platelet count, 18
platelets, 113, 116, 151
platform, 46
pleura, 7, 20
pleural effusion, 22
pleuritis, 22
pneumothorax, 2, 22
polar, 111, 148
policy, 27
population, 97, 102, 104, 123
portal vein, 22, 28, 35
positron, 78, 87, 104
positron emission tomography, 78, 87, 104
potential benefits, 99
precedent, 37
predictability, 200
preparation, iv, 48, 141, 201
prevention, 22
principles, vii, 1, 55, 62, 101
probability, 23, 35, 89, 92, 97, 100, 104
probe, 3, 9, 15, 16, 17, 18, 20, 21, 24, 25, 26, 35, 40, 41, 42, 43, 44, 45, 46, 58, 61
prognosis, 56, 100, 120, 121, 199, 207
proliferation, 97
prosthesis, x, 198, 201, 207, 209
protection, 64
prothrombin, 18, 113, 151
protons, 161
pulmonary embolism, 23
pulp, 186
purpura, 118, 119

Q

quality of life, 100, 199

R

radio, 55, 56, 57, 59, 61, 62, 63, 66, 68, 77, 106
radiography, ix, 173, 189, 190, 192, 194

radiotherapy, 39
readership, 120
reading, 141
real time, 24, 45
reality, 75, 81
recognition, 133, 162
recommendations, iv, 67, 69, 101
reconstruction, x, 80, 81, 83, 86, 90, 91, 93, 101, 106, 107, 138, 149, 150, 169, 170, 172, 176, 188, 197, 199, 200, 211
recreational, 122
recurrence, 3, 21, 23, 51, 53, 59, 66, 72, 138
red blood cells, 113, 151
reference frame, 40
reference system, 193
reflexes, 40
relaxation, 70
relevance, 86
reliability, 185, 207
remodelling, 88
repair, 143
requirements, x, 101, 197, 207
researchers, 95, 179
resection, 2, 55, 56, 58, 65
resistance, 16
resolution, viii, 24, 27, 40, 54, 79, 81, 84, 86, 96, 103, 155, 162, 176
respiration, 19, 37
response, 25, 26, 27, 50, 57, 67, 68, 77, 95, 125
restenosis, 90, 105, 106
rhythm, 83, 84, 106, 107
robotics, 48, 70, 73, 76
roots, 177
rubidium, 104
rules, 27

S

safety, vii, 1, 19, 21, 22, 27, 50, 52, 55, 64, 70, 94, 200
saturation, 161, 164
scar tissue, 95
science, 108, 179
scope, 82, 170

Index

second hand smoke, 99
seeding, 15, 20, 63
sensation, 207
senses, 16
sensing, 41, 47
sensitivity, 23, 26, 54, 84, 87, 90, 91, 97, 133, 156, 157, 158, 162, 167, 169
sensors, 47
sepsis, 19
severe stress, 87
shape, 5, 6, 15, 29, 50, 58, 207
shoot, viii, 79
showing, 41, 50, 92, 136
side effects, 2
signals, 25
signs, viii, 2, 117
simulation, x, 174, 176, 188, 190, 200
sinuses, 75
siphon, 166
skeleton, 174, 181
skin, 15, 20, 25, 29, 34, 35, 37, 42, 43, 97, 114, 152
sleep apnea, 129
smooth muscle, 139
society, 141, 148
sodium, 113, 151
software, x, 29, 31, 40, 41, 43, 45, 46, 71, 188, 192, 197, 199, 200, 201, 210
solution, 14, 17, 22, 61, 64, 200
specifications, 81
spin, 164
spindle, 138
spine, 140
splint, 37
splinting, 207
sponge, 5
stability, 74, 88, 199, 201, 209
standard deviation, 81
state, 36, 39, 76, 113, 118, 133, 151, 183
states, 36, 166
statistics, 129, 145
stenosis, 83, 84, 85, 86, 90, 91, 94, 96, 102, 103, 106, 125, 132, 134, 143, 150, 156, 157, 161, 162, 164, 165, 166, 171
stent, 90, 91, 105, 106, 201

sterile, 70
sternum, 35
steroids, 114, 152
stomach, 20, 22, 29
storage, 190
stress, 87, 100, 107, 200
stroke, 133, 135, 136, 144, 155, 158, 165, 168
structure, 22, 135, 155, 159, 176, 177, 181, 182, 186, 187
subacute, 95, 107, 116, 154
subdural hematoma, 116, 117, 118, 143, 153
substitution, 174, 188
subtraction, 143, 150, 157, 171
success rate, 36
succession, 163
superimposition, ix, 173, 176, 177, 179, 184, 185
suppression, 82
surgical intervention, x, 197, 200, 201
surgical resection, 3, 54, 57
surveillance, 164
survival, 3, 55, 57, 58
survival rate, 3
susceptibility, 27, 40
suture, 179
swelling, 114, 133, 152, 163
symmetry, 193
symptoms, 22
syndrome, 2, 89, 90, 112, 120, 133, 140, 142, 143, 146, 148, 187
synergistic effect, 17

T

target, viii, 3, 19, 21, 26, 27, 28, 29, 31, 36, 37, 41, 42, 43, 44, 45, 47, 52, 79
technician, 39, 198
techniques, vii, x, 1, 22, 31, 35, 37, 55, 62, 65, 71, 101, 131, 132, 161, 167, 176, 188, 197, 198, 199, 200, 207, 210
technology, ix, 3, 34, 36, 37, 40, 43, 47, 54, 70, 76, 80, 101, 103, 173, 174, 179, 180, 181, 182, 183, 184, 185, 188, 199, 200
teeth, 183, 199, 200
temperature, 3, 5, 7, 9, 17, 18, 58

222 Index

temporal lobe, 76
temporal lobe epilepsy, 76
territory, 87, 133
testing, 90, 100
tetralogy, 96
textbook, 211
thalamus, 136
therapy, vii, 1, 2, 3, 18, 26, 55, 56, 57, 58, 67, 69, 70, 75, 77, 107, 124, 128, 130, 192, 199
third dimension, 176
thrombin, 113, 115, 117, 151, 153, 154
thrombosis, 15, 22, 140, 164
thrombus, 114, 133, 152
titanium, 209
tooth, 199, 200, 201, 209
topical anesthetic, 122
toxicity, 15
training, 27, 47, 101
trajectory, 29, 31, 34, 41, 43, 44, 45, 46, 47, 122
transducer, 34, 35, 36
transformation, 35, 37, 43, 192, 195
transplantation, 3
trauma, viii, ix, 109, 112, 117, 140, 147, 150, 187
treatment, viii, ix, x, 2, 3, 16, 18, 24, 25, 26, 27, 28, 34, 36, 37, 38, 41, 50, 52, 54, 57, 58, 59, 61, 63, 64, 65, 66, 70, 75, 119, 124, 125, 131, 133, 142, 145, 146, 173, 174, 176, 177, 180, 185, 186, 187, 188, 192, 194, 197, 199, 211
tremor, 44
trial, 25, 56, 57, 58, 67, 84, 103, 105, 124, 125, 128, 129, 130, 131
trigeminal nerve, 71
trigeminal neuralgia, 75
turbulence, 161

U

ultrasonography, 67, 68

ultrasound, vii, 1, 67, 68, 70, 77, 89, 102
uniform, 5, 9, 26

V

vacuum, 37, 73
validation, 61, 189, 190, 193, 195
valuation, 77
variables, 180
variations, 185
vasodilation, 82
vasospasm, 123, 124, 144
vector, 187
vein, 22, 37, 93, 94, 106
ventilation, 39
vertebrae, 177
vertebral artery, 114, 151, 168
vessels, vii, viii, ix, 1, 5, 7, 15, 18, 20, 23, 36, 38, 92, 96, 109, 112, 113, 138, 147, 150, 151, 161, 167
vestibular schwannoma, 137, 146
videos, 120
viscera, 22
vision, 113, 150
visualization, 24, 28, 41, 75, 82, 86, 89, 104, 106, 200
vitamin K, 114, 152
vomiting, 133

W

walking, 113, 150
water, 24, 64, 81, 170, 176
weakness, 2, 116, 153
wear, 205
white blood cells, 113, 151
withdrawal, 20
workstation, 29, 40
worry, 209